The Primary Schizophrenia

A conference organised by
Research and Development for Psychiatry
and the Department of Health and chaired by
the Royal College of General Practitioners.

Second Edition

Edited by Rachel Jenkins and Vida Field

London: HMSO

ISBN 0 11 321979 2

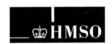

Pubished by HMSO and available from:

HMSO Publication Centre
(Mail, fax and telephone orders only)
PO Box 276, London, SW8 5DT
Telephone orders 0171 873 9090
General enquiries 0171 873 0011
Fax orders 0171 873 8200

HMSO Bookshops
49 High Holborn, London, WC1V 6HB
(counter service and fax orders only)
Fax 0171 831 1326
68-69 Bull Street, Birmingham, B4 6AD
0121 236 9696 Fax 0121 236 9699
33 Wine Street, Bristol, BS1 2BQ
0117 9264306 Fax 0117 9294515
9-21 Princess Street, Manchester, M60 8AS
0161 834 7201 Fax 0161 833 0634
16 Arthur Street, Belfast, BT1 4GD
01232 238451 Fax 01232 235401
71 Lothian Road, Edinburgh, EH3 9AZ
0131 479 3141 Fax 0131 479 3142
The HMSO Oriel Bookshop
The Friary, Cardiff, CF1 4AA
01222 395548 Fax 01222 384347

HMSO's Accredited Agents
(see Yellow Pages)

and through good booksellers

Printed in the United Kingdom for HMSO
Dd 302532 C150 9/96 9385 4231

Preface

This book is a revised second edition of the popular "Primary Care of Schizophrenia", based on one of a series of Department of Health conferences on mental illness and primary care. The conference was held in collaboration with the Sainsbury Centre for Mental Health (then called Research and Development for Psychiatry) which is an independent organisation committed to improving the quality of care of people with mental illness through research and development, and dissemination.

The first edition having rapidly sold out, the opportunity has been taken to ask the contributors to revise their chapters to take account of developments in the treatment of schizophrenia and of the more recent literature in the field. Some of the chapters have been completely rewritten, notably chapters 7, 11 and 12.

In a primary care led NHS, the utmost importance attaches to the primary care of one of our most difficult disorders to assess, diagnose and treat and we hope this book will be of assistance to primary care teams as they liaise with specialist health and social care services to provide the care their clients need.

Rachel Jenkins and Vida Field
August 1996

Contributors List

Dr Alastair Wright
Editor
British Journal of General Practice
Royal College of General Practitioners
14 Princes Gate
LONDON
SW7 1PU

Professor Julian Leff
Director
MRC Social and Community Psychiatry Unit
Institute of Psychiatry
De Crespigny Park
LONDON
SE5 8AF

Mrs Pam Jenkinson
President
Wokingham and District MIND
Berkshire

Dr John Reed
Special Adviser in Forensic Psychiatry
Department of Health
Wellington House
133–155 Waterloo Road
LONDON
SE1 8UG

Professor Digby Tantam
Professor of Psychotherapy
Department of Psychology and School of Postgraduate Medical Education
University of Warwick
COVENTRY
CV4 7AL

Dr Noreen Ring
Consultant Psychiatrist
Stockport Healthcare NHS Trust
STOCKPORT
Greater Manchester

Professor Geoff Shepherd
Head of Research
The Sainsbury Centre for Mental Health
134–138 Borough High Street
LONDON
SE1 1LB

Professor Peter Tyrer
Professor of Community Psychiatry
St Charles Hospital
LONDON
W10 6DZ

Dr Geraldine Strathdee
Consultant Psychiatrist
PACT Team
(Bethlem and Maudsley NHS Trust, Maudsley Hospital)
Denmark Hill
LONDON
SE5 8AZ

Dr Thomas Meredith Davies
Deputy Vice–Chairman, 1989–90
Royal College of General Practitioners
14 Princes Gate
LONDON
SW7 1PU

Mr John James
formerly General Manager
Kensington, Chelsea and Westminster Family Health Services Authority
88–94 Westbourne Grove
LONDON
W2 5XB

Mr Peter Clarke
Mental Health Services of Salford
Prestwich Hospital
Bury New Road
MANCHESTER
M25 7BL

Dr Hilary Hodge
NHS Executive
North West Regional Office
930–932 Birchwood Boulevard
Millennium Park, Birchwood
WARRINGTON
WA3 7QN

Dr Tony Kendrick
Department of General Practice
St George's Hospital Medical School
Cranmer Terrace
LONDON
SW17 0RE

Dr Rachel Jenkins
Principal Medical Officer
Department of Health
Wellington House
133–155 Waterloo Road
LONDON
SE1 8UG

Professor Michael Shepherd
Emeritus Professor
Institute of Psychiatry
de Crespigny park
Denmark Hill
London SE5 8AF

Joint-editor: (with Dr Rachel Jenkins)

Ms Vida Field
Reed Implementation Officer
Lambeth, Southwark and Lewisham Health Authority
1, Lower Marsh
London SE1 7NT

formerly
Policy and Information Manager,
Research and Development for Psychiatry
now The Sainsbury Centre for Mental Health
134–138 Borough High Street
London SE1 1LB

Contents

INTRODUCTION
Schizophrenia and the Primary Care Team: Prevention and Good Practice

ALASTAIR WRIGHT MBE MD FRCGP, Editor, British Journal of General Practice, Journal of the Royal College of General Practitioners, London.

The conference Schizophrenia and the Primary Care Team was sponsored by the Department of Health in collaboration with the Royal College of General Practitioners and Research and Development for Psychiatry to give general practitioners and team members an opportunity to discuss the often complex and urgent problems which schizophrenia poses and how these might be best dealt with in primary care settings. This book, which reflects the content of both the formal presentations and subsequent audience contribution made at the meeting, presents readers with many insights into schizophrenia itself; into the effects it has on patients and their families; into what can be done to help them now; and into areas worthy of further study—with emphasis on general practice and other primary care support networks.

Schizophrenia

GPs are at the front line in the diagnosis and treatment of mentally-ill people. Schizophrenia poses particularly difficult problems for them, for, unlike most illness, it distorts a person's ability to interpret reality and respond appropriately.

Changing Patterns in Management

Implications for primary care

The policy of replacing mental hospitals with a range of services provided locally means that patients with schizophrenia spend most of their time living in their own community. Although there still remains a clear requirement for the provision of acute beds and longer term 'asylum' and rehabilitation accommodation, hospital admissions have become briefer. This significantly increases GPs' involvement in patients' immediate and long-term care and in the provision of support for their carers. GPs now have:

increased contact with schizophrenic patients;

increased responsibilities;

increased need for liaison with local support services; and

1

increased potential to improve quality of care.

Liaison and responsibility

The GP will be able to reach a preliminary diagnosis in most cases of mental illness—including schizophrenia—but will pass the patient to a colleague in secondary care for confirmation, initiation of treatment, and development of a management plan which might involve shared care. Maintaining liaison with local psychiatric services is an essential part of maintaining continuity of care. To be effective, the GP and the primary care team must know about the availability and nature of local services, including day centres, hostels and the community psychiatric nursing service.

But, as authors of this book confirm, **increased liaison** means not only better links with consultant psychiatrists and psychiatric services. Collaboration with a wide variety of health professionals and community-based organisations and professions is essential: eg, with social workers, psychologists, local housing departments, the ambulance service, police, voluntary organisations and clergy representing local religious denominations.

Special consideration must be given to patients whose different racial and cultural backgrounds might make the diagnosis and management of their illness even more difficult. Health professionals need help to identify differences between values, behaviour and expectations accepted as normal in local 'indigenous' compared to 'minority' communities. These differences, if not recognised, can adversely affect assessment, management regimens, and thus the outcome of the illness. Liaison with representatives of ethnic groups in the area and provision of foreign-language materials can help overcome many problems—especially a patient's, or a family's reluctance to make or maintain contact with conventional health and support services.

Referral is thus not simply a matter of 'passing on' the patient to secondary care. Follow up and support are very much the province of primary care. The RCGP sees a cardinal role for a 'personal' doctor providing continuity of care and stable rapport with the patient wherever possible. This factor is especially important for schizophrenic patients—and often their carers—who have special difficulties in making and maintaining relationships.

Patients can behave in a bizarre fashion, but many of them are aware of their problems. Their worries are very realistically based: eg, about 'going mad'; about relapse; about social relationships and job prospects; and about care of their children and the risk of transmitting the illness to them.

Relatives can be devastated by the sudden onset of the illness in a previously healthy, young member of a family—perhaps the wage earner or a promising student. After their initial shock, they worry about the patient's future; about the impact schizophrenia will have on other family members—especially children; and about restrictions the illness will have on their own, the carers', lives.

Each patient and his or her family needs prompt, individualised attention. But certain core factors are common to all:

Carers need help with their anxiety; with their anger—which may focus on the patient, on the doctor, and/or, on health care team members; with their bereavement feelings of having 'lost' a loved relative; and, with their guilt. Could they have been responsible? Spotted it earlier? or, Coped better?

Patients need relief from distressing symptoms, and help with establishing realistic immediate and longer-term goals which address medical and social factors.

For these reasons alone, GPs have to work hard to provide efficient professional and sympathetic care. They and their primary care colleagues cannot shrink from these responsibilities.

The GP's role, as seen by the College, in addition to diagnosis, referral, emergency medication and admission is:

monitoring the patient's condition (including their physical health);

watching for relapse and side effects of medication;

acting as advocate for the patient or for the family.

Proposals for the Future

Research and education

Research into the epidemiology of schizophrenia in particular, and mental illness in general, should be vigorously pursued. Not only studies done by psychiatrists and in hospitals, but others by GPs and members of the primary care team working in primary-care settings. We need to know how doctors actually deal with mentally-ill patients and how we may best improve our skills in this major area of clinical practice.

Education should be woven into our daily work with patients: education appropriate for all members of the primary care team and where possible, our patients and clients. The College has already published information for primary care practitioners on depression[1], and schizophrenia[2].

Tackling 'Stigma'

Some GPs still prefer, and are expected to, concentrate on diagnosing organic disease, rather than psychological disturbance. Stigma attached to mental illness is still widespread[3]. The College would like to help improve this situation by working with our consultant colleagues and other members of the primary care team. In particular, we would like to develop close ties with the National Schizophrenia Fellowship—such as have already developed with the British Diabetic Association and similar bodies set up to provide non-medical support for chronic illness.

Developing long-term management protocols

A clinical priority of the College is to help improve the quality of care of chronic physical disease (such as cardiovascular disease, asthma and diabetes) by producing information for practitioners, organising study days with other health care professionals, and by encouraging the definition and development of clinical protocols for the major chronic diseases.

Most primary care practitioners are familiar with management protocols for hypertension and diabetes. Why not for depression and schizophrenia? The College would wish GPs to be more involved in the clinical care of schizophrenia as one of the major chronic diseases. Management protocols could facilitate this transition and help ensure high quality care.

The College would also welcome clarification of the roles of specialist and general practitioners so that the special knowledge and skills of each may be used most effectively. The wish is to encourage mutual respect and a strong working relationship between primary and secondary health care professionals and between doctors, patients and their families. We need and want to work together and we are willing to listen.

Community care is sometimes more of a slogan than a reality. Pressure to create really supportive community services must be maintained. The conference and this book show that there is no shortage of goodwill or good ideas in this field. I hope that future meetings will reveal carefully-documented and evaluated progress with many of them. But whatever developments emerge in the care of schizophrenia and other mental illnesses, there is no doubt at all that the GP will remain in the front line of action.

References

[1] Wright A. F., Royal College of General Practitioners. Depression: Recognition and Management in General Practice. London: RCGP 1993 ISBN 0 85084 180 1.

[2] Royal College of General Practitioners. *Schizophrenia Clinical Folder* London: RCGP, 1990.

[3] Sims A. The Scar that is more than Skin Deep. *British Journal of General Practice* 1993; **43**: 30–31.

Address for contact

The Editor, The British Journal of General Practice, Royal College of General Practitioners, 12 Queen Street, Edinburgh EH2 1JE.

1 Schizophrenia: Aetiology, prognosis and course

JULIAN LEFF, Director, MRC Social and Community Psychiatry Unit, Institute of Psychiatry, London

SUMMARY

Schizophrenia has to be defined by symptomatology because there is currently no laboratory test for the condition. It may well cover a diversity of conditions with differing aetiologies. However, heredity plays a substantial part in its transmission. Narrowly defined schizophrenia has a relatively constant incidence across the world affecting about 1 in 100 people. Brain imaging studies suggest a structural abnormality in a proportion of patients. Whatever the biological basis for the condition, patients are very sensitive to environmental stress, both acute (in the form of sudden events), and long-term (in the form of a tense atmosphere in the home). While maintenance anti-psychotic drugs reduce the relapse rate, they give only partial protection against stress. Helping patient and family to cope better with the everyday problems of living with schizophrenia confers additional benefit over and above drug treatment.

Introduction

Schizophrenia is almost a hundred years old. The idea of the illness was developed by Kraepelin[1] at the end of the last century, at a time when people were using a global concept of madness. He separated off schizophrenia from what he called manic depressive insanity. He did not actually use the term schizophrenia: that was coined some years later by Bleuler[2]. One of the first tests Kraepelin applied to this concept was to see if it worked in other cultures. This was very advanced thinking for the time. He took a trip to Java, had a look at the patients in the mental hospital there, and found to his delight that again, he could divide them off into patients he recognised as having schizophrenia and patients he recognised as having mania. He did not actually find any psychotic depressives in the hospital in Java, but that is another story.

His observations set off a whole line of international research into the cultural components of mental illness. This is not an exotic corner of psychiatry, but it occupies the centre field, because at the moment we have no pathological test which will tell you that a patient suffers from schizophrenia. In its absence, you have to rely on what the patient and the relatives tell you, and what people tell you depends very much on the culture from which they come. The questions of whether what they are saying is peculiar or abnormal has to be judged in relation to their background culture.

What causes schizophrenia?

In the last hundred years we have not made much progress in understanding schizophrenia. We are still at a stage in the development of the concept comparable to terms such as fever, or oedema (called dropsy in the 18th and 19th centuries) which are symptoms resulting from many different causes. Schizophrenia is still defined by its symptomatic picture which probably results from several aetiological factors.

Genetic Factors

General population vs family risk

One casual factor for which there is good evidence is inheritance. Part of the evidence is the increased risk if a member of the family is affected. The general population risk is one per cent: it is nine times higher if you have a brother or sister with schizophrenia, and 12 times higher if you have a parent with schizophrenia. If you are unfortunate enough to have two parents with schizophrenia, the risk rises to 40 per cent.

With the opening of the doors of mental hospitals, people with schizophrenia are increasingly marrying each other. It is quite difficult for someone with schizophrenia to marry a healthy person, because it is a grave disadvantage to have this disorder. Therefore, it tends to be patients who meet each other in hospital and at day centres who get married, and of course they then have a very high risk of having a child who will develop the illness.

Twins

Another approach to defining the genetic contribution to aetiology has been to look at twins[3]. There is a well established strategy of looking at the risks if twins come from the same egg, and share the same genetic material (monozygotic) or, if they come from two different eggs (dizygotic), in which case they are equivalent to siblings. Several studies have shown that if one twin has schizophrenia, risk for a monozygotic twin is between 25 and 50 per cent; for a dizygotic twin the risk is 10 per cent. So again, there is strong evidence for some genetic basis but by no means 100 per cent.

In considering the other 50, or even 75 per cent of monozygotic twins who do not develop the illness if their twin has it, geneticists have explored a number of possibilities, including incomplete penetrance: ie, the gene does not necessarily find expression in the illness. An alternative possibility and a growing focus of research interest is that there are *genetic and non-genetic forms of schizophrenia*. It may be that some of the disparate monozygotic twins are actually suffering from non-genetic schizophrenia. It has been suggested recently that non-genetic schizophrenia might arise from damage around the time of birth, and there is an increased incidence of perinatal complications in the early life of many schizophrenic patients[4].

Heredity and environment

Adoption studies represent another strategy for trying to sort out the different contributions of environment and heredity. Children who are adopted early from a schizophrenic parent (usually a mother) and taken to live with non-schizophrenic people, provide a very good way of looking at whether inheritance works its way through. If they are compared with children (of non-schizophrenic mothers) who were adopted early, there is a very big difference. The risk of schizophrenia is nil in the children of non-schizophrenic mothers; but 11 per cent for children of schizophrenic mothers. This latter risk is almost identical to the risk for a child brought up by a schizophrenic parent. In other words, we are seeing a very strong genetic component coming through, even when the environment is quite healthy[5].

Brain anatomy and physiology

The strong evidence for a genetic basis has led to a search for either anatomical or physiological abnormalities in the brains of people with schizophrenia. Unfortunately, there is not any clear cut answer to what the abnormality is. However, more precise methods of imaging the brain have been developed recently and reports have been coming out regularly of enlarged ventricles, indicating a reduction in the volume of the brain cortex. This abnormality has been reported in different areas of the brain[6]: the frontal lobes, the temporal lobes and even the cerebellum. However, there is a high proportion of schizophrenic patients whose brains look completely normal: only a small proportion are extreme on this measure of larger brain ventricles and smaller brain substance. A clear answer has not yet emerged from brain imaging, and the same is true of the psychophysiological studies.

Chromosome studies

More recently, there have been attempts using genetic linkage techniques to identify the particular chromosome on which the schizophrenic gene might lie. There have been two separate claims for different chromosomes, but as no one group has corroborated another group's findings, there is still confusion in the field. Of course, it is possible that two separate genes are responsible. The problem is that most studies are aimed at identifying a single aetiology, when in fact schizophrenia might be the final common pathway for many different aetiologies.

Epidemiological studies *{There is no mention of childhood influences}*

We now turn to epidemiological studies of schizophrenia, in particular the World Health Organisation (WHO) studies which have been very carefully

7

done, involving an enormous amount of work, and co-operation between different countries. One of the key studies, published in 1986[7], looked at the incidence of schizophrenia in a variety of different countries. Unfortunately, only one centre (Chandigarh in North India) was in the Third World. An attempt was made to include other Third World centres, but the work involved is very demanding. Research workers must pick up all possible cases of new schizophrenic illness within a certain time period. In a Third World country, with very limited psychiatric services, it is essential to screen the clients of traditional healers, people in prison, and vagrants. This is an enormous task which only one centre was able to do thoroughly.

Employing a broad diagnosis of schizophrenia, the incidence rates range from 11 to 35 per 100,000 population aged 15 to 54 years, which is the key period of risk (see Table 1.1).

Table 1.1: *The incidence of schizophrenia across cultures*

One year incidence rates per 100,000 population aged 15–54 years

Centre	Broad schizophrenia	Narrow schizophrenia	(%)
Aarhus	11.1	7.3	(66)
Moscow	23.9	12.1	(51)
Nagasaki	15.3	9.5	(62)
Nottingham	18.3	14.1	(77)
Chandigarh–urban	24.3	9.0	(37)
Chandigarh–rural	34.9	11.4	(33)

This threefold difference represents a statistically significant variation in the incidence. However, if a narrow definition is applied, (one which includes only patients with the first-rank symptoms elaborated by Kurt Schneider, another German psychiatrist[8] the rate becomes much more restricted (between 7 and 14). In particular, the exceedingly high rate in the rural area of Chandigarh shrinks down to the middle of the range of other countries. That is because only one third of the Chandigarh rural patients have nuclear, or first-rank-symptom schizophrenia.

The variation in range for narrow definition of schizophrenia is not significant, indicating a consistent incidence over a whole variety of cultures. This surprising result is not found with many diseases, even those known to be genetically determined. It means that if schizophrenia has a genetic basis, there must be a very regular gene pool throughout human populations, or, if there is a strong environmental component, it must be something which transcends major cultural differences between villages in North India, the City of Nottingham, Moscow and so on. This has really been a very important study in suggesting where we might look for aetiological factors. Certainly in the broad category of schizophrenia without first-rank symptoms, it would be advisable to look for environmental influences, particularly in Third World countries.

Stress and schizophrenia

Life events

We have reviewed the evidence for genetic factors, but this kind of work suggests there is also an environmental effect, and over the last 20 or 30 years we have got nearer to defining the environmental stresses which are linked with the origin of schizophrenia. One of them is life events, namely, sudden, often unexpected changes in the person's life circumstances. When these have been measured for people with schizophrenia, there is a clustering of life events in the three weeks before the onset of illness.

The first key study was conducted in Camberwell in South East London in 1968, on 50 patients[9]. Thirty–eight per cent of these patients experienced a life event independent of their illness in the three weeks before the onset of schizophrenia. This was a highly significant difference compared to the average rate over the whole three–month period before onset. A healthy group of controls reported only about 10 per cent having a life event reported in each three–week period before interview, so the patients showed a considerable excess.

These findings were confirmed by a WHO study[10] which included patients from a variety of cultures, and in most of them, there was a highly-significant clustering of life events in the few weeks before the onset of schizophrenia. This evidence supports the proposition that sudden stress can precipitate schizophrenia. That is not to conclude that they are the cause of the illness. It cannot be so because we all experience life events, but we do not all develop schizophrenia. It is however, reasonable to suggest that the genetic background gives rise to a latent tendency to develop schizophrenia which can be triggered off by environmental stress of this kind. *Does this refer to narrow or broad schizophrenia?*

Relatives' expressed emotion (EE)

Another form of environmental stress has been linked with the onset of episodes of schizophrenia: one which is more in the nature of long-term stress in the family and is associated with the concept of *Expressed Emotion (EE)*. This rather misleading term does not imply that all emotion is dangerous to patients, but three particular measures of relatives' emotional attitudes have been found to influence the outcome of schizophrenia. These are:

Critical Comments: Remarks or views expressed by the relative in an inter- *(medical)* view which are critical in tone or intent.

Hostility: Criticism is directed at the person rather than their behaviour in a rejecting way.

Overinvolvement: A too-intense emotional interaction with the patient, and/or over-protectiveness.

Patients who go home to live with relatives are more likely to relapse if the relative shows high criticism, any degree of hostility or a high rating on overinvolvement. By contrast, if the relative shows high warmth and does not express these negative emotions, the patient has a better outcome. It thus seems that relatives can influence the outcome of schizophrenia in a positive direction as well as a negative one. Studies have used these measures to create an *index of high Expressed Emotion* (high EE). The criteria are: six or more critical remarks in the interview; any degree of hostility; or a score of three or more on overinvolvement.

Many studies have now been done on high EE categorisation and relapse in schizophrenia across a large variety of different cultures and cities, including Chicago, Sydney, and Chandigarh[11]. Approximately 50 per cent of patients relapse over nine months if they live with a 'high EE' relative, compared with something between 12 and 25 per cent if they live in a 'low EE' household. A few studies have failed to show this association but, in the field of human research, these are really remarkably consistent findings and there is thus a strong suggestion that schizophrenic patients respond to their social environment just as indeed we all do. They are particularly vulnerable to acute stress and to more long-term stress.

The outcome of schizophrenia

Different perspectives: hospital vs general practice

A very important point to be grasped here is that there is a difference between the hospital view of outcome and the view from general practice:

In hospitals, we see the failures of community care; the patients who come back time and again; and we actually get a false view of the outcome of schizophrenia.

In the community, you see many more patients who never go back to hospital after the first onset.

In fact, the figure for a Western country like Britain is that, for a first onset illness, 25 per cent of patients will recover completely and will not have another illness for at least five years. That relatively good outcome is not obvious from the hospital view, because you do not see those patients again. The ones who stand out in your clinical practice are those who relapse every year. GPs in the community will have a different view because they see the patients with a much better outcome.

The few very long-term studies on groups of schizophrenic patients followed up in the community (about 15 or 20 years or more) tend to show a much better outcome than anyone taking a hospital view would have suspected. People like Manfred Bleuler in Switzerland[12], and Courtney Harding in America[13], have followed up cohorts of schizophrenic patients for several decades and found that a surprisingly high proportion recover, sometimes over many years, and live reasonably normal lives in the community. As many as 20 to 30 per cent have a satisfactory outcome, even though they might have had a disastrous beginning to their illness. This is a much more optimistic view than we would get from short-term studies in hospital.

The International Pilot Study of schizophrenia

There has been only one large outcome study of schizophrenia, again run by the WHO the *International Pilot Study of Schizophrenia*[14]. Samples of patients, collected in nine different centres in developing and developed countries, were followed up for two years. It is interesting that, despite the variation in cultures represented by the centres, about the same proportion of patients did very badly in each centre: about 10–15 per cent of patients never recovered from the illness and demonstrated psychotic symptoms throughout a two–year period. At the other end of the spectrum (for the percentage with the best outcome), dramatic differences appeared. Only six per cent of patients in Denmark had the best outcome; ie, recovered completely from the illness and did not have another episode in two years. By contrast, Agra in India and Ibadan in Nigeria stood out. There, over half the patients recovered and did not have another illness in two years. The five–year follow-up of this study shows the same pattern. These remarkable findings need explanation.

Factors influencing outcome

Which factors make the outcome better in these Third World countries? It is certainly *not* the quality of after care: the majority of patients have no continuing medication; most do not go back and see the psychiatrists; nor do they see a GP. They do *extraordinarily* well - not only in terms of their clinical outcome, but also in terms of their social progress. Patients from the three developing countries had the very best social outcome, with 13, 17 and 19 per cent showing severe social impairment, compared to over 25 per cent in the western countries. The **worst social outcome** was in Denmark which has possibly the **best community care** out of all the Western countries.

Relatives

So what is it—in the patients, in the society, or in the culture—which leads to such a good outcome? One possibility is the *attitude of relatives.* As explained above, Expressed Emotion has been measured in relatives across a variety of cultures. This has revealed a very wide variation in the proportion of relatives who are 'high EE'—ie, critical, hostile or overinvolved. On the west coast of America, in Los Angeles, two thirds of the English-speaking relatives have such attitudes—no different from Salford in the Midlands, Milan in Italy, or Cracow in Poland. By contrast, Mexican American relatives living in Los Angeles (interviewed in Spanish) showed only 40 per cent with high EE attitudes and North Indian city dwellers and peasant farmers showed 30 per cent and only 8 per cent respectively. These appears to be a spectrum which runs from the most to the least westernised cultures, with a differing degree of family tolerance for looking after schizophrenic patients.

Family structure

The varying degree of tolerance is partly due to differences in family structure: family life in rural India, for example, is mostly based on large extended families who give each other support; family life in Los Angeles, as in England, is disappearing. Not only has the extended family shrunk to the nuclear family; even the nuclear family is disappearing, and we are down to single parents. A high proportion of families are single-parent families, and in cases of schizophrenia, one often encounters a single, elderly relative—usually a woman in her 60s, 70s or 80s, and physically disabled herself—desperately trying to cope with a middle aged patient with schizophrenia. That situation is *never* seen in a Third World country where over 90% of patients live with their families and there will almost always be an extended family giving support; sharing the care of the disabled member.

Personal productivity

Attitudes to work differ. In Third World countries, there is not the same competitiveness or necessity for somebody to go to work and produce. *No one minds if the patient cannot be productive.* In addition, there are many positions in which relatively non-productive patients can be employed: in a rural area the patient can sit in the field and look after the corn and scare off the birds. In a rural society, there are unspecialised tasks quite suitable for handicapped patients which make them feel they are still contributing something to society.

Our problem in the West is, that somehow or other we have to make up for the families who have disappeared and create a supportive structure—not just for the patients—but for the single relatives who are often desperately trying to cope with schizophrenia. It is, of course, very expensive to create a network of professionals who act as a surrogate family, but we have to provide that form of support, because it is even more expensive to keep hospitalising patients.

Creating a professional support network

I will briefly describe the work we have done in trying to develop a professional support network, but it is necessary first to establish the nature of the protective factors which operation in 'high EE' homes. We noted that half the patients in such homes relapsed over nine months, while half remained well. The *good outcome* of the latter is accounted for by two protective factors:

(i)   *maintenance treatment with antipsychotic drugs* which reduces the relapse rate from nearly 100 per cent down to half that.

(ii)   *decreased social contact* between patient and the relative. If they can reduce contact the effect is as good as taking the drugs, lowering the relapse rate to about half, even if the patients are not taking drugs regularly.

If patients employ *both* protective factors, namely they take drugs and they reduce contact, the outcome is as good as in low EE homes.

Social protective factors

Given the inadequacy of drugs in completely preventing relapse in schizophrenia, the question arises of whether adding social treatment, which aims to alter the emotional environment in the home, to the drug treatment could further reduce the relapse rate. The social treatment we devised to help the families is a mixture of the following elements:

(i)   education about schizophrenia;
(ii)   helping the families to solve problems;
(iii)   improving their communication;
(iv)   dealing with their criticism and overinvolvement;
(v)   trying to cut down contact between the patient and the relative;
(vi)   expanding the social networks of the family, which have often shrunk because the family withdraws from social contact through embarrassment and shame; and
(vii)   lowering their expectations.

This last point (vii) involves teaching the family and the patient not to expect an immediate recovery. There is a prolonged convalescence period which can last one to two years before the patient returns to a more normal way of life[15].

Practical intervention programmes

It is very important that we reach out to these families in a way that professionals have been rather reluctant to do over the years. We provide a package of treatments in two forms:

(i)   *family sessions* in the home—which include the patients; and

(ii)   *a relatives group*, which excludes the patients but is run by professionals for the relatives, in a venue in the community.

We have run two different controlled trials of these forms of interventions:

(i)   We compared an experimental group (A) (who received the package of treatments) with a control group (B) (who received only routine outpatient care). We reduced Expressed Emotion and/or contact in three quarters of the (A) families, but it is important to note that, even in the control families (B) who received no family help, there was some spontaneous reduction in these factors[16].

(ii)   We gave family sessions alone, and also found that three quarters of the families (C) improved[17]. The alternative treatment offered was a group which relatives (D) were asked to attend. However, almost half the relatives did not come—even once—to the group! For those who came, the outcome in terms of change was as good as in group (C), but for those who did not, there were very small changes indeed (less than in the control group (B)).

Outcome

In terms of the outcome for schizophrenia, noting that almost all these patients were maintained on drugs, the relapse rate was reduced—from the 50 per cent expected without family help—to 8 per cent. The same reduction occurred with family treatment alone, and with the relatives' group for those who attended. The outcome for patients was very much worse if the relatives failed to attend the group.

We have concluded from this that it is *not enough just to offer a group:* the people who need it most will not come. *It is necessary to make the extra effort to visit the home and spend some time with the family as a whole.* In many cases, you can then persuade them to attend the group, but there will always be some families who will not attend. Some may have good reasons—like the mother who had agoraphobia. Sometimes the reasons are not so good—as with one couple who ran a pub together and said that they could not possibly leave it. We then held the family sessions in the pub outside of drinking hours!

The effect of the family treatments is to delay relapse over and above the delay possible to achieve with drugs alone. That is extremely valuable for patients, because it gives them a chance to re-establish their social relationships, their working abilities and their domestic skills. These forms of family help are not readily available, because they require a lot of skill. However, we are training nurses—including community psychiatric nurses—to use these kinds of intervention, which necessitate going out into the community and working with the families, in close co-operation with the GPs.

Conclusion

Schizophrenia is a complex disorder which, if treated promptly, and in a skilled manner can be controlled and allow the patient to resume a normal lifestyle. This may involve working with the patients and their families together or with the relatives alone—preferably in their own homes. The ability to reduce the frequency of high expressed emotion relationships between patients and their relatives and to allow recovery to take place gradually—over 1–2 years—is a key factor in success. Drug maintenance remains an essential part of management.

References

[1] Kraepelin E. Psychiatrie. 5th ed. Leipzig, Barth, 1896.
[2] Bleuler E. Dementia praecox oder Gruppe der Schizophrenien. in (ed. G. Aschaffenburg) Handbuch der Psychiatrie. Leipzig, Deuticke, 1911.
[3] Kringlen, E. Contributions of genetic studies on schizophrenia. In (eds. H. Häfner, W. F. Gattaz, W. Janzarik) *Search for the Causes of Schizophrenia.* Berlin, Springer–Verlag, 1987.
[4] Murray, R. M., Reveley, A. M., Lewis, S. V. Family history, obstetric complications and cerebral abnormality in schizophrenia. In (ed. H. A. Nasrallah) *Handbook of Schizophrenia,* Vol. 3. Amsterdam, Elsevier, 1988.

[5] Heston, L. L. Psychiatric disorders in foster home reared children of schizophrenic mothers. *British Journal of Psychiatry* 1966, **112:** 819–825.

[6] Shelton, R., Weinberger, D.R. X-ray computerised tomography studies in schizophrenia: a review and synthesis. In (eds H.A. Nasrallah, D.R. Weinberger) *The Neurology of schizophrenia.* Amsterdam, Elsevier, 1986.

[7] Sartorius, N., Jablensky, A., Korten, A. et al. Early manifestations and first-contact incidence of schizophrenia in different cultures. *Psychological Medicine* 1986; **16:** 909–928.

[8] Schneider K. Clinical Psychopathology. New York, Grune & Stratton, 1959.

[9] Brown, G . W., Birley, J. L. T. Crises and life changes and the onset of schizophrenia. *Journal of Health and Social Behaviour* 1968, **9:** 203–214.

[10] Day, R., Neilsen, J. A., Korten, A. et al. Stressful life events preceding the acute onset of schizophrenia: a cross national study from the World Health Organization. *Culture, Medicine and Psychiatry.* 1987; **11:** 123–205.

[11] Leff, J., Vaughn, C. *Expressed Emotion in Families: Its significance for Mental Illness.* New York, Guildford Press, 1985.

[12] Bleuler, M. (English trs.) *The Schizophrenic Disorders: Long-Term Patient and Family Studies.* New Haven, Yale University Press, 1978.

[13] Harding, C. M., Brooks, G. W., Ashikaga, T. et al. The Vermont longitudinal study of persons with severe mental illness. 1. Methodology, study sample and overall status 32 years later. *American Journal of Psychiatry,* **144,** 718–726.

[14] World Health Organization: *Schizophrenia: An International Follow-up Study.* Chichester, John Wiley & Sons, 1979.

[15] Kuipers, L., Leff, J., Lam, D. *Family Work for Schizophrenia: A Practical Guide.* London, Gaskell Books, 1992.

[16] Leff, J., Kuipers, L., Berkowitz, R. et al. A controlled trial of social intervention in the families of schizophrenic patients: two–year follow-up. *British Journal of Psychiatry.* 1985, **146:**594–600.

[17] Leff, J., Berkowitz, R., Shavit, N. et al. A trial of family therapy versus a relatives' group for schizophrenia: two-year follow-up. *British Journal of Psychiatry.* 1991, **157:** 571–577.

Address for contact

Professor Julian Leff, Director, MRC Social and Community Psychiatry Unit, Institute of Psychiatry, De Crespigny Park, London SE5 8AF.

2 The Real Life Experience of Schizophrenia from a Carer's Perspective

PAM JENKINSON, President, Wokingham & District MIND, Berkshire

SUMMARY

Schizophrenia, a mysterious and potentially devastating mental illness strikes apparently healthy young people without warning and knocks them (and their families) for six! Unless someone has experienced such an event personally, the full extent of the disturbance (and) disruption caused to all aspects of individual and family life and the despair engendered, is impossible to appreciate. This personal paper describes the burdens schizophrenia placed on my own family, turning me from a smiling 16 year-old schoolgirl into a bewildered and isolated 'carer' overnight, as my youngest sister, and later my brother, at the same age, succumbed to the disorder. Possible causes of schizophrenia, its effects on carers and suffers and methods of management are outlined. Early intervention by skilled health professionals; close liaison between them and the carers; varied support for the carers; active community-based management and rehabilitation programmes; and vigorous mental health education—made easily accessible to both sufferers and relatives are key points. As for carers themselves, the most important element is that they have somebody to help share the burden.

Background: Schizophrenia

What is schizophrenia? How does it start? What is the typical picture (see also Chapter 1)?

Schizophrenia comes 'out of the blue' as a total surprise and knocks the family for six! Most families are in a position of total ignorance about this serious mental illness. If one is only 16 or 17 when it strikes, as I was, it is particularly frightening. At that age, I assumed mental disturbance to be of psycho-social origin, and no teaching, however skilled, can dispel ideas that spring from immaturity. As my old Montessori tutor would say, "One cannot force mental growth." Shocked, I confused psychiatry with psychoanalysis and was resistant to the prospect of it—lest the psychoanalyst should find something wanting in me!

When I was young, I was always looking for an intellectual challenge—something I could not quite grasp. Schizophrenia has certainly given me that.

After 33 years, I remain puzzled. Nobody fully understands the illness, and it has puzzled everyone since Bleuler[1] brought the attention of the medical world to this mysterious form of dementia which attacks the apparently young and healthy, 'out of the blue'. We have clues about it: like Saint Paul, we 'see through the glass darkly'. There is something hereditary about it, and it is very much associated with environmental stress.

When I was well into my twenties and was, one day, observing my sister and brother, both of whom suffer from schizophrenia, it suddenly dawned on me that they suffered from a physical condition—*"a stress-related biological disorder"* as Dr Ian Falloon describes it[2].

I would have described my sister as a very normal little girl. Her primary school report described her behaviour as 'exemplary'. In her second year at grammar school, she received a school prize for "progress"—not brilliant then (for good or ill, I was the 'brilliant' one), but of exemplary behaviour and progressing well. She was just 15 when this happy picture changed and she began to display schizophrenic symptoms. Is schizophrenia, then connected with puberty?

In her case, initial symptoms included social withdrawal, social refusal, and eventually, refusal to leave the house. Her behaviour did not become wildly disturbed until some time later. Professionals described this process as 'insidious onset followed by acute psychotic breakdown'. For me, as a carer, I recall, that from the Autumn of 1962, I entered a nightmare existence. My father was terminally ill, and life consisted half of visiting him in hospital and half of coping with the disturbed situation at home. I am afraid that there was not much fun in my 18–year old existence. Mother?

Carers and caring

In order to gain insight into the real life experience of schizophrenia from the point of view of a carer, one could do worse than to glance through the pages of the carer's old family photograph album—especially if the carer, like I do, keeps the photographs in chronological order. What rapidly becomes obvious is that at some point normal life came to a sudden stop. In my case, the observer sees:

> August 1962: Pam aged 16; in school uniform, having just passed 'O' levels; smiling

> Next
> August 1967: Pam, aged 21; with friend at Summer School; smiling.

What happened during and to the five intervening years? Why are there no smiling photographs? **Schizophrenia had struck the family. All normal life had ceased.**

I was only 16 when schizophrenia struck my family and I became a carer. Mature or not, carers are all confused, and few realise in those early days that schizophrenia is an illness like any other; that the first port of call is the GP who will refer the patient to a consultant psychiatrist who, in turn, will almost certainly prescribe medication and perhaps electro-convulsive therapy (ECT).

The chief difference between the real-life experience of schizophrenia from the carer's point of view—as distinct from that of the medical professional—is that the carer's point of view is entirely personal. He or she is concerned with the way in which their personal life is affected by the burden of caring. Sometimes (and particularly in the case of women) one's professional life can be affected as well—in terms of inability to accept career advancement due to the competing demands of caring for a dependent relative. The carer in most instances is also thrown back upon personal resources.

Doctors, nurses and social workers receive, in varying degrees, rigorous training and have professional support systems. In general, carers 'learn as they go along'. Professionals start from a sound information base. Carers start, usually from a point of total ignorance and bewilderment, and gradually acquire skills, knowledge and coping strategies.

A point about carers! However ignorant, however frightened they might be, carers cannot just abandon their relatives. They are determined to do what is best for them. When I was very young, I gave permission for my sister to have electro-convulsive therapy—as recommended by the consultant—because, despite the controversy which rages around that treatment, I believed it was best for her.

The most important element in any caring situation is that there is somebody to share the burden. Carers who are unsupported and alone can collapse under the strain. The experience which led me to this conclusion was entirely personal. I cared for a sick mother—sharing the caring equally with a very capable and sympathetic brother. This arrangement worked perfectly for several years until my mother died. The patient received first class care and was extremely happy. My brother and I were both happy and neither felt over-burdened. The message is therefore 'SHARE THE CARING'- and if no other relative is available, a friend or neighbour may be willing to come to a satisfactory arrangement.

The family burden

I put studies on the 'back-burner', temporarily, because I wanted to give priority attention to my father. I found my situation curiously ambivalent. The message I picked up from my school was that they disliked me and that I was responsible for my sister's illness; that they wanted to get the schizophrenia out of the school as quickly as possible; but they very much wanted me to stay so that they could get academic honours out of me. Some professionals describe this as a double-bind message. I hurriedly left the school, making sure that they got no academic honours but, in due course, I went to Cambridge where I spent an enjoyable time.

My father died in 1964 and, about that time, my brother, then aged 15, also started to display schizophrenic symptoms. I have heard Dr Timothy Crow say that if schizophrenia was entirely psychosocial in origin, siblings would react to their disturbed environment by becoming ill at the same time. But this does not happen. Instead, they become ill at a similar age. When my brother became ill as well, I thought that life had become an everlasting nightmare.

'Some are born to endless night' says Blake in his poem, *Auguries of Innocence*. I certainly believed I was.

Social workers were involved with the family by this time, but they took a long time to initiate medical contact and treatment. Psychotherapy or talking treatment, has no effect upon acute schizophrenia. If one has the benefit of early intervention treatment for schizophrenia—as practised by Dr Ian Falloon[2] Professor Julian Leff[3], and Dr Max Birchwood *et al*[4]—the trauma of compulsory admission under the Mental Health Act is often averted, but way back in the 1960s there was no such enlightenment, The guru of popular psychiatry was R D Laing, *and families were blamed, not helped.* ⟶ Was this because of a perceived connection with factors in early life?

Good practice

(i) Early intervention

I wish that the models of early intervention set up by Ian Falloon in Buckingham and by Max Birchwood in the West Midlands could be extended to other areas of the country. These models involve training GPs to pick up early signs of schizophrenic illness and to initiate low-dose drug treatment before one is faced with a full-blown episode. I do not want families to experience the situation I had with my brother. When I finally called our two family practitioners to admit him to hospital under the Mental Health Act, on grounds of his own health, he was too psychotic to recognise them. "Who are you?" he asked. They had treated the family for years.

Early intervention can save money on NHS acute beds and also result in less trauma for families[5]. I did not like seeing my relatives admitted to the mental hospital, and they did not like going in. The hospital was miles from our home, and we would all have preferred home treatment. That is not to deny that some beds must be kept for mental illness.

I have taught groups at the National Schizophrenia Fellowship (NSF) and they regard many of my views as idealistic. In their experience, approved social workers do not exist; it is very difficult to obtain an acute mental illness bed; and even more difficult to get any information from doctors and other professionals involved in the care of their relatives.

STRENGTHENING THE LOBBY

(ii) Relatives need a strong voice

The question of professional carers confiding in the relative(s) for instance, is a thorny one. The NSF has made representations to the Royal Colleges on the issue—pointing out that anyone in a caring role needs full knowledge about the diagnosis, prognosis, treatment, and aftercare of the patient. This is the pragmatic view. Opposing this is the view, held by some professionals, that the medical records of adults are confidential in all circumstances.

Having worked for the NSF and run the Schizophrenia Training Consultancy for years, in 1992 I set up the National Alliance of the Relatives of the Mentally Ill—in order to strengthen our lobby.

(iii) Long-term outcome

After 33 years of being involved with schzophrenia, I have settled my brother and my sister independently, in their own flats, in the community. That was not easy!

I had looked after my sick mother until she died in 1985. In the latter days of her illness, I actively prepared my brother and sister for her death and for coping with life without her. As a result of this preparatory work, my mother's death was nothing like the trauma it might have been for them, and they adjusted well to her loss and their new situation.

I was determined that their standard of living would at least resemble my own, and that I would not be over-involved or critical (see chapter 4), but neither would I lose touch. As a result, a limited relationship is maintained, and I can be called upon when needed. For example, my sister recently asked me to discuss her anaemia with her GP and to make sure that iron was the right treatment for her. She had refused to have a gynaecological examination, so I told the GP that this suspicion was due to her schizophrenia and did not cast any slur on him. I also told him that our mother had suffered from sideroblastic anaemia, an inherited condition, and that it might be advisable to test my sister for this. He found the interchange very helpful. Relatives can be a source of useful information as well as recipients of it.

Schizophrenia in the family has a long-term effect upon one's professional life as well as one's personal life. I doubt that I would have been much interested in mental illness had I not been so closely affected by it. Given other circumstances, I would probably have been a literary critic or the headmistress of a girls' school: people tell me that I am the 'headmistressy' type! Instead, I decided to devote my talents to mental health. I worked very hard for many years—providing support groups and training, but the crying need is for **practical** help.

The Wokingham Crisis House

My Relatives Support Group was greatly in favour of setting up a Crisis House so I set one up in April 1991 as soon as I could get a lease on a house under the auspices of our local Mental Health Association (MIND). The House does not restrict itself to sufferers from schizoprenia and their relatives; it deals with all mental health problems but schizophrenia is by far the commonest diagnosis of those who use the facility. The Crisis House is managed by a Committee of twelve people—half of whom have recovered from mental health problems and half of whom are carers. It is totally consumer run. No professionals are involved.

The Crisis House provides support and sanctuary for people who are relapsing with schizophrenia but who are not ill enough to warrant hospital admission. It also provides temporary sanctuary for suffers who are well enough for discharge from hospital but who are waiting for their community care arrangements to be finalised. Both services are extremely useful because timely asylum can prevent acute breakdown and the necessity for hospital admission, and temporary (or stopgap) asylum gives the professionals assuming responsibility for the individuals's community care the time to think through the arrangements carefully without the person having to occupy a psychiatric bed while this is done.

Some of the crises which we deal with are extremely acute and include people who are referred to our House as a 'Place of Safety' under Section 136 of the 1983 Mental Health Act. We enjoy an excellent relationship with the local Police. Some of our clients, by contrast, are working through a life crisis and may need sanctuary for some weeks or months. Such people may be referred by local General Practitioners, social workers, community psychiatric nurses and the Samaritans. The Crisis House is an extremely low-cost facility since all the crisis work is carried out by volunteers and the local community gives enormous support in terms of everything that is needed to run the House. Such a model could be followed in other areas—thus enhancing provision for the primary care of schizophrenia and relieving the burden on carers.

HOSPITAL BEDS ARE STILL NEEDED

Many people are unaware of the provisions of the 1983 Mental Health Act. Recently, I had to read the Act over the telephone to a GP who was reluctant to come out and admit, under a Section, a young man who, suffering from schizophrenia, was behaving violently towards his mother. In such circumstances, the individual does not have to give consent to admission. Under Section 4 of the Mental Health Act, the nearest relative may apply for the patient's urgent admission, compulsorily, to hospital, on grounds of his own health or safety, or with a view to the safety of other people.

This is not to suggest that the majority of schizophrenia suffers are dangerous. Very few are. Nor is it true that chonic schizophrenia sufferers place a disproportionate burden upon GP services. It is the *neurotic* population who take up more of the GPs' time. Not only do they frequently take up medical time; they are going to the wrong shop! Boredom, marital difficulties and dissatisfaction with life are not cured by medicine. New interests and the service of others are the cure. In contrast, schizophrenia is a treatable condition which usually responds well to medication and psycho-social support but some hospital beds for those who relapse will always be needed.

Benefits of mental health education

An ideal outcome

Mary had been attending my Relatives Support Group in a helping capacity when schizophrenia hit her family 'out of the blue'. She has three grown-up children: two have been diagnosed as having schizophrenia; one has been described as having 'schizoid features'. Her eldest daughter, a qualified nurse serving in HM Forces, became ill first. Mary was contacted, without warning, and told that her daughter was suffering from schizophrenia and would be invalided out of the army. She received first-class treatment in a military hospital.

Mary was only too well aware of what 'aftercare' can mean—having attended my relatives' group and listened to the experiences of others. I recommended the Richmond Fellowship, and her daughter went straight into one of the rehabilitation hostels on discharge from hospital. From there she was able to resume low-stress nursing in a private geriatric hospital; and from there, well-recovered and on minimal maintenance medication, she was able to resume full-scale professional nursing in an NHS hospital. In order to avoid the high expressed emotion situation which can develop if a sufferer lives with close family (see chapter 4), Mary arranged for her daughter to live in supported lodgings with a sympathetic landlady.

This description is an ideal outcome, and I am now helping Mary to achieve a similar outcome with her other children.

What are the elements in a good outcome?

A good outcome depends on three main factors:

First: the carer is intelligent and energetic—eg, a trained teacher and nurse.
Second: initial treatment is speedy and of high quality.
Third: the carer has access to expert information.

Psychiatric rehabilitation

The existence of rehabilitation programmes is not common knowledge. Many carers stumble upon such information only after years of trauma. Psychiatric rehabilitation must be immediate and entered into as part of an ongoing treatment programme. When this happens, chronicity is avoided. Medication should be reduced but not discarded, so that the sufferer can resume work. There needs to be—as Dr Roger Morgan says—'an atmosphere of stimulation[6]'. What frequently happens to schizophrenia sufferers on discharge from hospital is that they just return to their families, sit back (or lie in bed) and do nothing. Professor John Wing[7] says that the very worst thing for schizophrenia suffers is to sit about doing nothing all day. With good GP services, early intervention and minimal hospitalisation, sufferers can keep (or quickly resume) jobs, and thus maintain quality lives as equal citizens.

Psychiatric rehabilitation has to be sensibly structured—allowing for increasing levels of independence as suffers recover and progress. Some sufferers will experience relapse(s) if the programme is too vigorous. Support is needed at all stages.

Conclusion

After 33 years of experience, I now feel comfortable in describing schizophrenia as *'a stress-related biological disorder with a genetic component which usually responds well to anti-psychotic medication and ongoing psychosocial support.'* All these elements must be taken into consideration in the provision of good psychiatric services.

References

[1] Bleuler, E. Dementia praecox oder Gruppe de Schizophrenien in (eg G. Aschaftenburg) Handbuch der Psychiatrie. Leipzig, Deutike, 1911.

[2] Falloon, I. R. H., Boyd, J. L., McGill, C. W. et al 1985 Family management in the prevention of morbidity of Schizophrenia: Clinical outcome of a two year longitudinal study. *Archives of General Psychiatry* **42**, 887–896.

[3] Leff, J., Kuipers, L., Berkowitz, R. et al, 1985 A controlled trial of social intervention in the families of schizophrenia patients: two year follow up. *British Journal of Psychiatry* **146**, 594–600.

[4] Birchwood, M., Smith, J., Macmillan, F. et al, 1989. Predicting relapse in schizophrenia: the development and implementation of an early signs monitoring system using patients and families as observers. *Psychological Medicine* **19**, 649–656.

[5] Pringle, J., 1970. A case of schizophrenia. Letter to *The Times*, May 1970 (available from the National Schizophrenia Fellowship, 28 Castle Street, Kingston upon Thames, Surrey KT1 1SS).

[6] Morgan, R., 1981. Psychiatric Rehabilitation. National Schizophrenia Fellowship.

[7] Wing, J. Personal Communication made at a training session for NSF co-ordinators.

Address for contact

Mrs Pam Jenkinson, President, Wokingham and District, MIND, Community Mental Health Centre, Station House, Station Approach, Wokingham, Berkshire RG11 2AP.

Further reading

F. N. Watts and D. H. Bennett (eds), *Theory and Practice of Psychiatric Rehabilitation,* Wiley: Chichester, 1991 (2nd edition)

A Lavender, F. Holloway (eds) *Community Care in Practice,* Wiley, Chichester, 1988

P. Jenkinson, *No Drugs. No ECT. How I overcame Clinical Depression.* STC Publications, 1990 (available from STC, 69 Shepherds Lane, Bracknell, Berkshire RG12 2BU).

3 Mental Health Policy

DR JOHN REED, Special Adviser in Forensic Psychiatry, Department of Health, London

Introduction

In the wake of the White Paper "Caring for People"[1] published in 1989 the Department of Health sponsored a series of conferences about mental illness and the primary care services, with a view to identifying ways of improving prevention, detection and management by the primary care team. This chapter looks at mental health policy including developments since "Caring for People" and considers the impact of schizophrenia on primary care.

Current Mental Health Policy

Present mental health policy in England and Wales is based on two simple principles. First, that care should be given as locally to where a person lives as is reasonably possible and secondly that it should be available in the least restrictive conditions that are compatible with the safety of the patient, of those caring for him and of the public at large. The system that provided mental health care mainly in large asylums distant from where patients lived grew gradually during the 19th and early 20th centuries. The 1808 Asylum Act gave local authorities permissive powers to build mental hospitals and the 1845 Lunatic Asylum Act obliged authorities, within three years, to provide asylums. However, even as the asylum system developed there were moves away from it.

The first domiciliary Crisis Intervention Service was started in the 1880s and the first out-patient clinic in 1889. In 1918 the Board of Control (then responsible for the mental health service) suggested that early treatment units in general hospitals would be helpful in speeding recovery. Clinicians found that better results could be achieved with less reliance on in-patient care and the move back to local care was reflected in the 1930 Mental Treatment Act which allowed treatment without certification and greatly promoted out-patient care.

It was against this background of steady change that the major tranquillisers were introduced in the mid–1950s. The effect of these combined events was dramatic. On 31 December 1954 there were roughly 150,000 patients in mental illness hospitals and units, by 1969 there were just over 116,000. These dramatic changes in hospital population and in clinical practice naturally commanded great interest at the Ministry of Health, as it then was. An influential paper by two Ministerial officials (Tooth and Brooke)[2] set out the changes in hospital population to date and predicted a further decline in the number of beds used despite the continued occurrence of people with long-term mental health needs.

Now in 1993 there are some 50,000 beds in NHS hospitals, but recent research has shown that although the number of beds for mentally ill people in NHS hospital and units has declined there has been a corresponding increase in the number of beds provided by other agencies such as the voluntary sector and local authorities so that for some ten years the total number available has remained broadly steady. The policy consequences of these changes was first set out by the then Minister for Health, Enoch Powell[3], in his famous "water towers" speech in March 1961. The policy was set out in detail in the 1975 White Paper "Better Services for the Mentally Ill"[4] and was reaffirmed in the White Paper "Caring for People" where it was described as a "civilised and humanitarian" policy. The basic requirements of the policy are that health authorities should develop comprehensive services for mentally ill people as locally to their homes as is possible and that this should be done in association with local authorities and voluntary organisations. More recently, the White Paper "Health of the Nation"[5] has identified mental illness as one of the five key areas for health gain. It sets three targets:–

> to improve significantly the health and social functioning of mentally ill people.

> to reduce the overall suicide rate by at least 15% by the year 2000 (from 11.0 per 100,000 population to no more than 9.4)

> to reduce the suicide rate among severely mentally ill people by at least 33% by the year 2000 (from the life-time estimate of 15% to no more than 10%.

All targets which are very relevant to those suffering from schizophrenia.

It has never been the intention of policy to move to a solely community based service. The aim is for a service providing a proper balance of in-patient treatment and community care to meet the varying needs of mentally ill people. It is important to recall that closure of hospitals has never been a primary aim of policy; a hospital should not close until there has been proper reprovision of the services that it provided. The change from a distant, large, institution based service to a local service offering both hospital and community care is a major one, not likely to be achieved without some problems and the need for "finetuning" in implementation. For instance, recent research has shown a significant unmet need for longer term in-patient care in conditions of security below the highest levels[6].

Maintaining Long Term Care

Rightly much concern has been expressed about failures of the mental health services to ensure that mentally ill people receive the care they need once discharged from hospital. At best this can lead to unnecessary relapse and at worst to homelessness, dereliction and entry to the criminal justice system, at times as a result of terrible acts of violence. Several inquiries into failures of care have highlighted many problems in ensuring adequate care [7,8]. To help promote more effective care the Department of Health has developed a range of initiatives. Assertive action to maintain contact with patients who have left hospital is essential to good mental health care and reduces relapse and offending[9]. Since 1991 DH has been promoting assertive follow-up through the Care Programme Approach[10] which requires that all patients of the specialist psychiatric service have a clearly identified care plan, a key worker responsible for co-ordinating its delivery and regular re-assessments. In addition, before discharge from hospital patients must have been assessed as set out in the Discharge Guidance[11] (1994) and not discharged unless and until their doctor is confident that their needs can safely be met in the community. Those most at risk of violence, self-harm or neglect must be included in a supervision register[12] which acts as an aid to prioritisation and as a checklist of the most vulnerable. Subject to completion of the passage of legislation additional legal powers will become available allowing for formal "aftercare under supervision" of some categories of patients.

Mentally disordered offenders

It has long been recognised that a number of mentally disordered people become detained in the criminal justice system. There are two objectives in ensuring that mentally disordered people in the criminal justice system receive the mental health care they need. Firstly, to ensure care and treatment by health and social services rather than in the criminal justice system for those who meet the criteria for admission to hospital under the Mental Health Act 1983. (Studies conducted by Gunn et al [13, 14] show that some 30% of prisoners have a mental disorder and that 2% have a serious (psychotic) mental illness requiring transfer to hospital.) Secondly, to provide mental health care in the prison system to "the same standards of health care as those provided by the NHS"[15] for the much greater number of people who do not meet the criteria for transfer. (Gunn et al more recent study found that 10% of the sentenced prison population required mental health care in prison. A further 6% (mainly those with personality and sexual disorders) needed a therapeutic community within the prison system.)

Ensuring care in the NHS for those who need it has been hard to achieve. Recognising the difficulties Ministers in Department of Health and the Home Office, at the end of 1990, established a review of services for Mentally Disordered Offenders which completed its work in mid 1992. The review set out five guiding principles [Annex A] which underlie its recommendations and which, for the first time, set out a clear ethical framework for the service. It made 276 recommendations and published seven volumes of reports [Annex B]. Ministers in both Departments have accepted that the review sets the general framework within which, as resources allow, they wish to see services develop.

References

[1] Department of Health (1989) *Caring for People: Community Care in the Next Decade and Beyond*. London HMSO
[2] Tooth, C.G. and Brooke, E.M. (1961) Trends in the Mental Hospital Population and their Effect on Future Planning. *Lancet* **i** 710–713.
[3] Powell, E. (1961) Address to the National Association for Mental Health in Emerging Patterns for the Mental Health Services and the Public. London, NAMH

[4] Department of Health and Social Security (1975) *Better Services for the Mentally Ill*. London, HMSO Cmnd 6233

[5] Department of Health (1992). The Health of the Nation: *A strategy for health in England*. London, HMSO Cm 1986

[6] NHS Executive (1995). High Security Psychiatric Services: *Changes in Funding and Organisation*. London, Department of Health

[7] Department of Health and Social Security (1988). Report of the Committee of Inquiry into the Care and Aftercare of Miss Sharon Campbell. London, HMSO Cm 440

[8] Department of Health (1994). Report of the Inquiry into the Care and Treatment of Christopher Clunis. London, HMSO

[9] Tyrer P., Morgan J., Van Horn E., Jayakody M. et al (1995) A randomised controlled study of close monitoring of vulnerable psychiatric patients *Lancet* **345** 756–759

[10] Department of Health (1990). *The Care Programme Approach for People with a Mental Illness referred to the specialist psychiatric service HC(90)23/LASSL(90)11*. London, Department of Health

[11] NHS Executive (1994). *Guidance on the discharge of mentally disordered people and their continuing care in the community HSG(94)27*. Heywood, Department of Health

[12] NHS Management Executive. *Introduction of supervision registers for mentally ill people*. Heywood, Department of Health

[13] Gunn J., Robertson G., Dell S., Way C. (1978). *Psychiatric aspects of imprisonment*. London, Academic Press

[14] Gunn J., Maden A., Swinton M. (1991). Treatment needs of prisoners with psychiatric disorders. *British Medical Journal* **303** 338–341

[15] Home Office (1991). *Custody, Care and Justice*. London, HMSO

Annex A

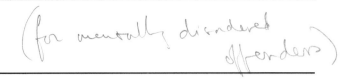
(for mentally disordered offenders)

Guiding principles—patients should be cared for:

i.   With regard to the quality of care and proper attention to the needs of individuals;

ii.   As far as possible, in the community rather than in institutional settings;

iii. Under conditions of no greater security than is justified by the degree of danger they present to themselves or to others;

iv.   In such a way as to maximise rehabilitation and their chances of sustaining an independent life;

v.   As near as possible to their own homes or families if they have them.

Annex B

Review of health and social services for mentally disordered offenders and other requiring similar services (the "Reed" review)

These reports may be purchased directly from HMSO. They are not available from the Department of Health or the Home Office.

Volume 1 Final Summary Report (Cm 2088)
ISBN 0-10-120882-0 (November 1992)
£12.40

Volume 2 Service needs (report of the community, hospital and prison advisory groups and a Steering Committee Overview) (January 1993)
ISBN 0-11-321551-7
£24.00

Volume 3 Finance, staffing and training (reports of the finance, staffing and training advisory groups) (January 1993)
ISBN 0-11-321552-5
£18.00

Volume 4 The academic and research base (reports of the academic and research advisory groups) (January 1993)
ISBN 0-11-321553-3
£6.50

Volume 5 Special issues and differing needs (report of the official working group on services for mentally disordered offenders with special needs) (January 1993)
ISBN 0-11-321554-1
£12.50

Volume 6 Race, Gender and Equal Opportunities (February 1994)
ISBN 0-11-321700-5
£7.00

Volume 7 People with Learning Disabilities (Mental Handicap) or with Autism (February 1994)
ISBN 0-11-321701-3
£22.00

HMSO publications are available from:–

HMSO Publication Centre (Mail, fax and telephone orders only)
PO Box 276, London SW8 5DT

Telephone orders   0171-873-9090
General enquiries   0171-873-0011
Fax orders   0171-873-8200

4 Schizophrenia: What Treatment is available?

DIGBY TANTAM, Professor of Psychotherapy, University of Warwick
NOREEN RING, Consultant Psychiatrist, Stockport Healthcare NHS Trust

SUMMARY

In acute episodes of schizophrenia, florid symptoms dominate the clinical picture but it is the deficit symptoms which are more important over the long term. Neuroleptics (major tranquillisers) are the treatment of choice for florid symptoms, although practical aspects of care are also important during periods of disturbed behaviour. The long-term use of neuroleptics, whilst it may prevent relapse in many patients, is not enough to prevent the accumulation of deficit symptoms. For the patient in the community, a minimal-effective-dose prescribing policy should be combined with psychosocial intervention and support of carers.

Background

Although as many as a quarter of the inceptions of schizophrenia result in complete recovery, the burden of schizophrenia is due to the remainder which become chronic, recurrent, or both. It is often helpful to consider the symptoms of chronic schizophrenia as falling into two groups:

(i) *florid symptoms*, which include hallucinations, delusions, motility disorders, and thought disorder. These are also associated with acute schizophrenia and are the dominant symptoms during relapse. They do not always remit completely with treatment, in which cases they will persist even after acute behavioural disturbance has passed; and

(ii) *deficit symptoms*, which include lack of emotional expressiveness, reduction in social speech, social withdrawal, lack of initiative, and a lack of emotional engagement in the lives of other people. These symptoms are particularly troublesome between relapses and, because they are much less likely than florid symptoms to disturb other people, they may come to medical attention less readily. However, evidence from outcome studies suggests they are more important for the long-term social outcome.

V. much what Colin has
(8/12/98)

33

Treatment of florid symptoms

Neuroleptic drugs

The mainstay of the treatment of florid symptoms is the prescription of neuroleptic drugs ('major tranquillisers', 'antipsychotics'). These all appear to have a dopamine-blocking action in common, and they most probably act by affecting the activity of dopaminergic mesocortical and mesolimbic neurons although other mechanisms of action have not been excluded. Individual neuroleptics have been championed as being more effective than others for all patients, but this impression has not been borne out by clinical experience. Some patients do seem to respond better to one drug than another, though, and it is worth enquiring about this possibility in those who are relapsing, so that the preferred drug may be used. If this information is not available, the choice between drugs is dictated by patient acceptability and ease and reliability of administration. Patient acceptability is especially important in long-term treatment where lack of compliance can be a major problem.

Classification and properties

The most useful and simple classification of neuroleptics is:

(i)   low potency (hundreds of milligrams used)
(ii)   high potency (less than 50 mgm used)

and each of these may be used as

(iii)   oral or
(iv)   depot preparations
(v)   atypical neuroleptics

Low-potency neuroleptics tend to cause more atropinic side-effects such as dry mouth, blurring of vision, constipation, sedation, and complications in overdose.

High-potency neuroleptics have more prominent extra pyramidal side-effects: dystonia and dyskinesia (involuntary, usually buccopharyngeal movements or involuntary gait or postural disturbance), akathisia (involuntary restlessness and agitation), akinesia (lack of movement), and tremor. The neurological side-effects of low-potency neuroleptics are probably masked by their intrinsic anticholinergic action, and the prevalence of delayed (tardive) extrapyramidal effects (notably tardive dyskinesia) is the same as that with the high-potency drugs. The delay in diagnosis of tardive dyskinesia means that it takes some time to evaluate this side-effect when a neuroleptic is newly introduced.

Idiosyncratic effects such as hepatotoxicity and neutropenia occur, albeit rarely, with all neuroleptics.

Atypical antipsychotics

An atypical antipsychotic has been defined by Kerwin[1] as an effective neuroleptic which has "a wide therapeutic ratio for its antipsychotic effects and extra-pyramidal side-effects, such that these are not seen at clinically effective doses".

Clozapine, which causes fewer extra-pyramidal side-effects and may be more effective in refractory cases causes a ten-fold higher incidence of neutropenia and its use is currently restricted to treatment resistant patients, treated by psychiatrists registered with a monitoring service organised by the manufacturers. Risperidone (a central $5HT_2$ and D_2 antagonist) has been found to be effective in treating positive and negative symptoms of schizophrenia while reducing the risk of extra-pyramidal symptoms.

Depot preparations are given by intramuscular injection. Depending on their chemical preparation and rate of release, effective blood levels can be maintained for between three days (clopenthixol) and a month (haloperidol decanoate; pipothiazine palmitate). They were introduced to ensure compliance, but are not always preferable to oral agents (see Table 4.1). Under research conditions, tablets are associated with a lower relapse rate compared to depot preparations—possibly because patients who receive information about their medication are able to increase the dose, as necessary, to deal with an upsurge of florid symptoms (see also psychosocial education below).

Table 4.1: *Relative advantages and disadvantages of oral depot neuroleptics*

Neuroleptic drugs	
Oral preparations	Depot preparations
Advantages	
Flexible doses	Patient is monitored when injection given
Patient has some control of dosage	Compliance monitored
Prescription monitored with each new supply	
Disadvantages	
Poor compliance	Patient discomfort
	Administration costs

Non-neuroleptic drugs

Anticholinergic drugs such as procyclidine or benzhexol may be used to counteract acute extrapyramidal side-effects. However, they have side-effects of their own. Taking them, for example, increases the risk of tardive dyskinesia, unwanted sedation and dependence. Routine prescription is thus not recommended, except to prevent acute dystonia—a most frightening side-effect. Acute dystonia most commonly occurs a few days after starting a young patient on a high-potency or high-dose neuroleptic for the first time.

Diazepam is occasionally used as an effective adjuvant to neuroleptics in the sedation of highly-disturbed patients with acute psychoses, but it is not normally indicated and is not an effective antipsychotic.

It should be noted that antidepressants can worsen psychotic symptoms.

Non-pharmacological treatment of florid symptoms

Although as many as 40 per cent of patients have persistent florid symptoms despite comprehensive drug treatment[2], there are few alternative treatments.

Electro-convulsive therapy (ECT) can be effective, but is rarely used because psychotic patients rarely consent and because public and professional opinion is strongly against any element of coercion in its use.

Leucotomy has neurological consequences which make it unacceptable nowadays.

Psychological treatments rarely help patients with florid symptoms of schizophrenia. Those which have been used include confrontation of delusions, psychodynamic psychotherapy, cognitive therapy and distraction techniques for auditory hallucinations. Only the last two have any enduring benefit for a significant number of patients. Auditory hallucinations are among the commonest florid symptoms, but their interference with everyday activities is sometimes overlooked. Music played into the dominant ear from a portable cassette recorder, or just plugging the ear, can be effective.

Persistent positive symptoms are often refractory to drug treatment. Much of the force of these symptoms derives from their distressing content. Patients may have the delusion that their brains have been removed, or hear voices telling them that they are the anti-Christ. Cognitive therapy can effectively reduce the frequency or associated distress of these persistent symptoms in many cases. Various strategies are used, but they all involve an invitation to the patient to consider the evidence for and against the possibility that their belief is mistaken, or that the voice is misleading. Skill and ingenuity is required to put these strategies into practice, particularly if emotional pressure on the patient—which can make their symptoms worse—is to be avoided[4].

Treatment setting

Prompt treatment with neuroleptics can shorten the duration of illness and prevent the development of aggressive impulses, self-neglect, or disturbed behaviour. However, protracted illness occurs in 10 per cent of new cases of schizophrenia, and special care is required in a much larger percentage to counter the adverse psychosocial consequences of an acute episode. In the past such care was usually provided by admission to hospital which has several theoretical advantages:

Patients in a first episode can be thoroughly investigated to detect those who have a physical disorder; they receive asylum from the sometimes hostile responses of others to their illness; they are looked after by expert carers; and their carers obtain respite.

In practice, these advantages are often offset by the disadvantages of being uprooted and placed in a new, challenging, and socially impoverished setting. Behaviour might deteriorate away from the moderating influence of the patient's customary environment. Nurses, although expert in the illness, cannot compete with the carers' knowledge of their charges. Any advantage gained by lifting the carer's responsibilities is often outweighed by their worries about the absent patient. Forgetting about the patient is even worse, since families may find it more stressful to have the patient return home.

Extra care is always required during psychosis. Acute psychosis is associated with an increased risk of violence, of self-harm, of self-neglect, and of disturbed behaviour in **some** patients. Hospital admission will continue to be necessary for very disturbed people, but more forms of alternative care are now available. These include day care during crisis, home care by community nurses, and 24–hour help lines. In some areas, accommodation in the community can be provided during a crisis which provides some respite and, possibly, some supervision, without the complete break from normal living caused by hospital admission.

Treatment of deficit symptoms

Neuroleptic drugs sometimes worsen and sometimes improve deficit symptoms, because deficit symptoms can be reactions to unadmitted florid symptoms; eg, social withdrawal can result from intrusive hallucinations or delusions. The atypical neuroleptics are said to be more effective in ameliorating deficit symptoms, but the evidence is inconclusive. (Clozapine etc.)

The mainstay of treatment of deficit symptoms is psychosocial, rather than pharmacological intervention. Deficit symptoms such as lack of initiative and social unresponsiveness can be overcome by overtures from other people. In situations of social impoverishment, social withdrawal and lack of social response are amplified. Such deprivation can lead to the bizarre or stereo-typed behaviour associated with 'institutionalism', and such behaviour is not shown only by long-term institutional residents: mild examples are more common and more easily overlooked in community settings.

Forced social involvement carries with it the risk of failure and usually involves emotional demand, which can provoke relapse. However, active, but task-orientated involvement (eg, in work or in domestic activities within shared accommodation) can be designed to increase the likelihood of social involvement and of task attainment. 'Assertive community outreach' and the structured activities of many hospital hostels are two applications of this approach.

Social involvement in structured work and residential situations is one element of rehabilitation, which also includes training, or retraining in living skills. Rather than putting patients through a routine 'rehabilitation programme', the programme or 'care plan' should be fitted to suit the patient.

Care programmes

The Care Programme Approach has been adopted to improve the delivery of services to people with psychological disorders. It aims to ensure that services are appropriate to meet needs, and that patients do not slip through the services net. The detail and formality of care programmes will vary according to the complexity and severity of patient's problems. People with schizophrenia who come into contact with mental health services will normally be reviewed at a special meeting, following a multidisciplinary assessment of health and care needs. If there is serious concern about the patient's danger to themselves or others, this review may lead to the patient's name being placed on a supervision register. There are drawbacks to this, as no additional resources are identified and no powers conferred by placing patients on a register, and there is a danger of stigmatising patients.

The care programme normally consists of a written care plan; a clear indication of the member of staff with responsibility for making the plan work (the 'keyworker'); details of other staff involved with the patient; an indication of how agencies and professionals will work together; provision for consultation with the patient him- or herself and with any concerned family or friends; and a date for review of the plan once it has been in operation. General practitioners may participate in the review meetings, as well as being members of the team with responsibility for delivering the care plan. Because of the GP's time commitments it is unlikely that the GP him– or herself would wish to be the keyworker, however involvement in care planning seems increasingly important as more GPs share care with psychiatrists.

Prevention of schizophrenia

Medication and psychoeducation strategies

Primary prevention of schizophrenia is still beyond reach, although evidence continues to accumulate that perinatal injury or viral infection is associated with the later development of schizophrenia. However, relapse and, to a lesser extent, deficit symptoms can be greatly reduced, even prevented ('secondary' and 'tertiary' prevention: see also Chapter 1).

Prolonged treatment with neuroleptic drugs considerably reduces relapse rate, but at the cost of long-term side-effects, including aggravation of the lack of initiative and diminished emotional response which are socially debilitating.

Intermittent prolonged medication alone has not been a success. Even when the relapse rate can be reduced, considerable morbidity occurs as a result of the greater anxiety and depression patients experience. *Continuous treatment at lower doses,* has been more successful, with several researchers finding little change in relapse rate, but a significant reduction in side-effects[3].

Flexible medication regimens combined with psychoeducation strategies (see Table 4.2) which involve patients and their carers offer several advantages. Patients and carers usually learn more about the nature and effects of schizophrenia and the drugs used in its treatment. They are taught to recognise early warning signs of relapse (insomnia and unexplained anxiety or depression are prominent ones) which precede frank psychosis, and so can restart (or modify) therapy before the illness becomes self-sustaining and more refractory to medication.

Table 4.2: *Elements of a psychoeducation programme for patients and carers (long-term management of schizophrenia)*

Element	Content
Diagnosis and prognosis	What is wrong What effect(s) will the 'illness' have The term 'schizophrenia' is used only if the patient or relative would be helped by having a precise diagnosis
Use and effects of medication	Importance/benefits of compliance
Side-effects of medication	Recognition/management of unwanted side-effects
Model of schizophrenia	Arousal
Early warning signs of relapse	Patient/carers may be given a list of symptoms to watch for
Pathway back to treatment	What to do when relapse is in the offing

Psychoeducation strategies, such as those outlined in Table 4.2, are welcomed by many (but not all) patients and particularly by their carers. They help patients and carers gain greater control of the illness, and so of their daily lives, and offset the hopelessness a diagnosis of schizophrenia can engender.

The most effective prolonged neuroleptic strategy now available is to continue treatment after remission for all but a selected group of patients in their first episode. After a period of 'psychoeducation' of the patient and any involved relatives, patients whose symptoms have completely remitted and who are not in any obvious danger of relapse may be treated according to a dose-reduction protocol. The elements of this include gradual withdrawal of unnecessary medication, monotherapy with whichever neuroleptic is the patient's choice, and establishment of a rapid-response procedure in the event of threatened relapse. Once these conditions are satisfied the dose of neuroleptic can be progressively, although slowly, reduced until the patient is beginning to have prodromal symptoms or to be taking extra self-prescribed medication. At that point, the dose should be increased to its immediately preceding level. Further dose-reduction may be tried after a period of stability (eg 3–6 months).

A note of caution

Primary depression (ie, depression not associated with overt or unadmitted relapse) is not uncommon in schizophrenia and usually responds to anti-depressants. In view of their potential for increasing psychotic symptoms, these should be used only when relapse has been ruled out.

The caring network

Depression and anxiety are over-represented in patients with schizophrenia and in their carers. Schizophrenia is a perplexing illness, and it is difficult for parents or other relatives not to think that some of its manifestations are 'put on' by the patient, out of spite or indolence. Living with a young man whose behaviour is erratic is often frightening for older parents, who may feel powerless to influence their son's behaviour. Parents carry much of the burden of the care of patients with schizophrenia and, unfortunately, often find professionals are unresponsive to them in crises which are too easily labelled a 'social problem' (see Chapter 2).

Overstressed parents are more likely to show the characteristics of 'high expressed emotion' (EE)[5] which is associated with an increased relapse rate. The obverse of this is that people with schizophrenia who live in 'low EE' households relapse less than those who live alone. Considerable attention has been paid, therefore, to improving family coping styles which can reduce EE. This can be effectively done in parent groups (although these appear not to be acceptable to some parents) as well as in family therapy (see also Chapter 1).

Prevention overview

Social stress model

Both relatives and patients benefit from a systematic model of schizophrenia designed to help them:

(i) predict the effects of life-style and behaviour on schizophrenia, and

(ii) plan how best to cope with effects of the illness.

One useful approach is to explain that schizophrenia affects a person's ability to manage social situations: people interacting with someone who has schizophrenia must therefore make special social efforts. Everyday situations, especially changes, are more stressful than they are for the average person, and people with schizophrenia have a greater tendency to use coping methods, such as social withdrawal, inappropriately.

This 'social stress' model emphasizes four aims for the management of schizophrenia by patients and their relatives:

(i)   Stress monitoring
(ii)   Stress management
(iii)   Coping strategies
(iv)   Social skills training

Some potential stresses, such as social situations which require a high level of interpersonal understanding and influencing skills, can and should be avoided. The avoidance of all stress, however, is both impossible and undesirable. Exposure to manageable stress increases tolerance to future stress; avoidance of stress diminishes the ability to cope. Adverse response to stress can be diminished by medication; by undemanding social support; and by social withdrawal used judiciously so as to avoid social disruption. Patients and relatives need therefore to be taught about stress monitoring, using 'early warning signs'; to be given more flexibility over medication; and to be encouraged to tolerate social withdrawal, if used appropriately. Specific training in coping with unavoidable social demand such as job interviews can be useful. Social skills training can make patients more independent and more assertive.

Carers benefit from learning how to monitor their own stress levels; and medication, social support, and time-out can all help them cope with the socially—and emotionally—demanding task of living with schizophrenia. Those who are not coping well might find that training in different, less emotionally-arousing strategies improves their situation.

Marginalisation

Despite the best efforts to prevent it, schizophrenia can cause irreversible social breakdown—often as a consequence of disturbed behaviour which is perceived as wilful rather than involuntary[6]. There is an increasingly tendency for men with schizophrenia to abuse alcohol or drugs, and this can exacerbate florid symptoms. The disturbed and sometimes violent behaviour which can result is particularly likely to lead to a censorious response, because it is apparently avoidable. About 30 per cent of the growing number of homeless people living on city streets in the developed world have mental illnesses, and many of them also abuse alcohol and drugs. Theirs is a dangerous and unhealthy life, with restricted access to basic health care. Their treatment needs are often simple but unmet: eg, dental care, detection and treatment of physical illness, and the prescription of neuroleptic medication[7].

The GP's contribution to care of patients with schizophrenia

The expectation that patients with schizophrenia will have most of their treatment outside hospital means that GPs and other primary care providers are becoming much more directly involved. Shared care between hospitals and GPs is being developed, but much remains to be worked out. The GP is well placed to offer long-term continuing care in a familiar, accessible and non-stigmatising environment. He/she may have the advantage of already having developed a relationship with the patient or the family. The GP can also offer preventive health care to this group of patients who are known to have increased rates of physical illness. There is a need to develop a pro-active approach to identify and maintain contact with patients suffering from schizophrenia. This can be achieved by collaboration between GPs and community psychiatric nurses. Negative symptoms such as social withdrawal and lack of initiative may prevent them from seeking help and they might otherwise only present at times of crisis.

Conclusion

The treatment of florid symptoms of schizophrenia is important. It needs to be extended to all psychotic patients, including those out of touch with health care systems because of homelessness or other social marginalisation. Early treatment is highly desirable to prevent social deterioration. Hospital admission is not always necessary and, in general, social disruption should be kept to the minimum necessary to ensure the patient's adequate care, and to protect the patient and others from aggression or the consequences of disturbed behaviour.

In the long-term, the treatment of deficit symptoms is probably more important. Medication should be kept to the minimum needed to prevent relapse, and psychosocial intervention given centre stage. Patients can be usefully involved in monitoring their own relapse potential, and in collaborating with the doctor in titrating their neuroleptic dose against this. This collaboration should form part of a wider programme in which the patient, the doctor, and other staff participate in planning work, accommodation and leisure, so as to increase the patient's social contacts, independence, and active involvement in keeping him or herself well. Carers who live with patients should also be involved in some of these interventions to reduce the burden on them and to increase the social richness of the home environment without increasing emotional demand.

Monitoring the patient's progress and providing assistance with problems as they arise will often be carried out by a non-medical key-worker. Most of the doctor's time may go on the supervision of medication. However, the doctor's particular authority is likely to make him or her especially able to provide support and advice at key moments. The involvement of the GP in the community and in the family makes him or her well qualified to make this contribution to the holistic care of the patient with schizophrenia.

 integrated

Address for contact

Digby Tantam, Professor of Psychotherapy, Department of Psychology and School of Postgraduate Medical Education, University of Warwick, Coventry CV4 7AL.

References

[1] Kerwin, R. (1994) "Atypical neuroleptics", *British Journal of Psychiatry* **164**, 141–148.

[2] Harrow M., Carone B. J., Westermeyer J. F. The course of psychosis in early phases of schizophrenia. *American Journal of Psychiatry* 1985; **142**: 702–707.

[3] Marder S. R., Van Putten T., Mintz J., Levell M., McKenzie J., May P. R. Low and conventional–dose maintenance therapy with fluphenazine decanoate: two-year outcome. *Archives of General Psychiatry* 1987; **44**: 518–521.

[4] Kingdon D., Turkington D., and John C. (1994) "Cognitive behavioural therapy of schizophrenia", *British Journal of Psychiatry* **164**, 581–587.

[5] Kuipers L., Bebbington P. Relatives as a resource in the management of functional illness. *British Journal of Psychiatry* 1985; **147**: 465–470.

[6] Fadden G., Bebbington P., Kuipers L. The burden of care: the impact of functional psychiatric illness on the patient's family. *British Journal of Psychiatry* 1987: **150:** 285–292.

[7] Tantam D. High-risk groups: the homeless and ethnic minorities. *Current Opinion in Psychiatry* 1991; **4:** 295–303.

5 The Management of Schizophrenia in the Community: What Services do we need?

GEOFF SHEPHERD, Head of Research, The Sainsbury Centre for Mental Health

SUMMARY

The management of schizophrenia in the community is a difficult and complex task. It demands services which will pay as much attention to the management of disability as to the treatment of symptoms. Managing disability in schizophrenia depends upon offering sufferers the maximum opportunities for social reintegration, while at the same time ensuring they receive a degree of "shelter" which is appropriate to their individual needs. This means providing a range of residential facilities, day care, and community support which will cover the entire spectrum of functions previously served by the mental hospital. In addition, effective community services also require good coordination and mobile staff resources who will take services to patients, rather than waiting for them to come to the services. GPs have a crucial role to play in monitoring, delivering and developing good community services, and it is hoped that they may be able to develop close working partnerships with a variety of mental health professionals to achieve their common aims.

Background

The course and outcome of schizophrenia is strongly influenced by a range of social and environmental factors. In particular, both cross-culturally and within cultures, outcomes can be shown to be closely related to opportunities for social reintegration [1,2]. 'Community care', with its emphasis on helping people with serious mental illnesses integrate into the community and live as 'normal' a life as possible should, therefore have much to offer in the successful management of this disorder. GPs clearly have a central role to play in this process.

Community Care

The concept of 'community care' is still controversial. Its critics point out that the notion of 'community' is vague and that the 'community' cannot be expected to 'care' by itself. To succeed, there must be an adequate range of resources present in the community to support people with long-term mental illness, otherwise the burden will simply fall on to families, GPs, etc.

Successful community care therefore means developing what Leona Bachrach has called 'functional equivalents' to the mental hospital[3]. She argues that it is not possible to do away with the mental hospital unless we understand very clearly the complex range of functions that hospitals provided. Thus, we need to develop an adequate range of services in the community (residential, occupational, social, medical) not just provide somewhere to live. This means transferring funds out of hospitals and health authorities and into social services and other community agencies. This has proved extremely difficult.

In addition to *moving resources*, community care also means considerable *changes in staff attitudes*. Many mental health professionals still expect to deliver care primarily in fixed sites (hospitals, outpatient clinics, day services), they expect patients to attend for treatment and to be motivated to receive it. People with severe schizophrenia may fulfil none of these expectations, and those in the greatest need are often those who have to be seen in their own homes and whose motivation is the worst. We therefore need to develop much more flexible attitudes, both about *where* care is delivered and *who* is seen to have priority. Before I sketch out what is required to deal with these problems let me begin with a brief look at the nature of schizophrenia.

Schizophrenia: The nature of the problem

The problems experienced by people with schizophrenia will be familiar to many GPs and primary health care teams. In addition to the presenting symptoms, both 'positive' (eg, hallucinations and delusions) and 'negative' (eg, lack of motivation, apathy and social withdrawal), there may also be a range of adverse personal reactions and social handicaps. In the former category we would include denial, and feelings of depression, hopelessness and despair about the future. These are all understandable reactions to the occurrence of a severe and disabling mental illness (indeed, they may also occur as a reaction to severe physical illness such as heart disease or diabetes). Their presence underlines the importance of simple counselling and the provision of a stable, trusting relationship were the patient can be helped to come to terms with the condition and make as positive an adjustment as possible. GPs as well as other health professionals can make an important contribution to this process. Without a good relationship, it may be impossible to deliver the formal medical aspects of care (eg, medication) and, as with the management of other long-term conditions, compliance with treatment plans may depend on a mutual understanding of the shared goals of care.

The GP may also become involved with the social handicaps of schizophrenia, eg, the reactions of family, friends and employers. Providing simple information and support can then be of direct benefit to the patient, helping them receive more positive social support and enabling them to maintain jobs and relationships that would otherwise be at risk of breakdown.

Maintaining adjustment in the community is often very difficult for people with schizophrenia because of their sensitivity to life events and life change. None of us can avoid life events and we all have to learn strategies for coping.

People with schizophrenia find it very difficult to deal with life events which entail major changes to established routines. Although the events themselves may be quite positive (eg, moving to new accommodation; starting a new job or relationship), many patients lack both a flexible repertoire of coping strategies and good networks of social support. There has thus been considerable interest in efforts to help patients improve their coping skills and expand their social supports[3,4]. It is not yet clear how successful those interventions are likely to prove, but in the meantime, life events are useful 'markers' of periods of increased stress and risk of relapse.

As indicated in the introduction, the most important factors influencing long-term outcome in schizophrenia are probably not those associated with symptom control (although this is certainly important, see Chapter 4) but those associated with long-term social adjustments. Several studies, both of individuals and groups, have demonstrated the relative independence of symptomatic and social outcomes. Thus, some patients show a poor outcome in terms of symptoms, but a relatively good outcome in social terms. Conversely, a greater number of patients show quite good symptomatic outcome, but remain socially rather disabled. This separation of 'symptoms' and 'functioning' means that we cannot assume that treating symptoms successfully will necessarily improve functioning. A separate range of services is needed, which is especially targeted to preserve the patient's ability to function in the community. Examples of such services are described below.

Community Support:
Options for the long-term mentally ill

Residential Services

Garety[5] and Morris[6] in their excellent reviews of residential services both emphasise the need for as wide a range of residential options as possible. Some patients manage perfectly well in flats and 'bed-sits' with minimal supervision; some need regular—perhaps daily—staff visits; others may require 24-hour, intensive supervision. The range of needs is enormous and it is a challenge for each area to develop facilities which span this spectrum. This means close working together of statutory and voluntary agencies over long periods of time.

In recent years, several important issues have emerged regarding **residential care** which are worth noting:

(i) **A tendency to underestimate the need for highly supervised, permanent places.** Misplaced optimism in the late sixties and early seventies suggested that the problems observed among schizophrenic patients in hospital were simply *caused* by the hospital environment and were not related to any intrinsic features of the disorder: ie, if patients could be maintained outside hospital, their problems would disappear. Unfortunately this assumption has turned out to be largely incorrect. Caring for people with schizophrenia in community settings has shown that many of their *problems are intrinsic* to the disorder - although they may be exacerbated by environmental factors.

Transfer to the community is therefore not a magic solution for improving functioning.

Patients can therefore show signs of 'institutionlisation' in community settings (eg, group homes and hostels). Even in their own homes. They do not always improve and, as a result of rehabilitation, become able to move on to less and less supervised accommodation. Of course, this is not to say that patients never change or progress, but it does cast doubt on the traditional approach to providing residential care where the emphasis is on moving through a fixed series of residential facilities of gradually decreasing levels of dependency. This can place undue stress on the patient. It is much better to provide permanent accommodation, with high levels of supervision which are flexible, and which take account of fluctuating levels of need. It may then be necessary to *move the staff* around the network from time to time, rather than the patients.

The question of exactly how much accommodation of different types is required by each district is difficult to specify. However, an attempt has been made to produce some general guidelines based on an epidemiological analysis of need by Wing (1992)[7]. These figures have to be interpreted according to local circumstances, particularly taking into account levels of social deprivation. Thus, the need for sheltered and supported housing may be three times greater in a deprived inner city area, compared with a relatively prosperous shire county. Needless to say, *actual* levels of provision are substantially below the recommended guidelines.

(ii) **Questions of quality.** What constitutes good *quality* residential care? Which kinds of environment are likely to be associated with positive change and which are likely to lead to deterioration? It is probably easier to specify the features associated with poor environments (eg, lack of stimulation, lack of individualised care, 'block' treatments, rigid routines, etc) than it is to define high quality care. *'Quality'* must be defined multidimensionally and must take into account everything from physical facilities, to staffing levels and management practices.[8]

The key to defining high quality care is respect for the uniqueness of each individual and their right to a high 'personalised' package of care and a personalised environment.

The problem with assessing quality of care is not just defining it. We must also address the question of how to *monitor* quality effectively and how to ensure that poor quality services, once identified, are changed and improved. This is a very difficult task, given the range and variety of providers in the community, but monitoring must proceed on the basis of some kind of personal inspection. While local authority inspectorates remain in their infancy, networks of local GPs may have an important role to play, making statutory agencies aware of problems they encounter through their contacts with residential homes. This responsibility cannot fall solely on GPs, but they are well placed to be aware of such difficulties.

(iii) **Young, 'new' long-term patients.** A few young *'new'* long-term patients have now emerged who cannot be managed in the traditional range of group homes and hostels. Most of them have a diagnosis of schizophrenia and show high levels of both positive and negative symptoms which are highly resistant to drug treatment. These patients are the most difficult of the young schizophrenics and they require a very specialised setting to meet their needs. Bennett[9] coined the term *'ward-in-a-house'* to describe such a facility which contains the best features of high quality hospital care (eg, expert use of medication, skilled nursing care, individualised programmes) combined with the best features of high quality community care (eg, small size, homely setting, easy access to shops). Several 'ward-in-a-house' or hospital hostel developments have been established, and the results gathered over the past 10 years are promising [10,11] although they are clearly not a panacea. Districts could use a specialised facility of this kind to deal with their most difficult cases.

Day care services

Day care services are as important as residential care in the management of people with schizophrenia in the community. Day care is usually provided in one of two forms: (a) occupational ('work') activities; or (b) social/therapeutic activities.

a. 'Work' activities

Work has traditionally consisted of fairly routine industrial tasks (eg, sub-contract packing and assembly) and this has generally been provided in industrial therapy units in hospitals, or day centres in the community run by local Social Services departments. However, both the nature and organisation of work services is now changing.

New work projects are being established which aim to provide *'real work'* in the form of goods and services relevant to local needs. These projects are often run like small businesses, with the emphasis on providing a realistic work atmosphere and high levels of contact with the public and community[12]. The providers are usually voluntary agencies such as Richmond Fellowship, British Institute for Industrial Therapy (BIIT), or local MIND groups. These small, local organisations have the advantages of flexibility and not being tainted with traditional 'institutional' attitudes.

The staff often have a background in commerce, rather than in the 'caring' professions, and this means that they bring a different set of attitudes and expectations. They are more interested in what people *can* do, rather than what they *can't*, and this can provide a healthy antidote to the emphasis on pathology and disability which is often prevalent among mental health professionals.

There is also considerable interest in various forms of **placement schemes** where the individual is placed in an open employment setting, usually part-time, and given extra help and support to enable him or her to maintain the position. There are many different versions of such schemes, but all rely for their success on careful selection and preparation of the patients, combined with equally careful preparation and support of employers. Again, GPs may be asked to form part of the back-up services to support the individual and reassure the employer.

Problems arise in many work projects about the payment of **realistic wages**, since most of the 'employees' retain their social security benefits. Nevertheless, it is sometimes possible to pay people a certain amount in goods or 'in kind' without it affecting their benefits. Many patients are prepared to work for very little financial reward if the work itself is interesting and is seen to improve confidence and self-esteem. People may also earn a small amount per week on 'therapeutic earnings' without affecting their benefits if their GP is prepared to indicate that part-time work will benefit their mental health and rehabilitation.

b. Social/therapeutic activities

Social support for long-term patients in the community has also seen considerable changes in recent years. In the past, support was often provided in the day centres, and usually entailed keeping patients 'entertained' in a rather passive, chronic, 'sick' role. (Alternatively, they might be exposed to a never-ending diet of 'therapy'). Recently, these patterns have begun to change and modern social centres tend to be run more on the lines of a social 'club', with *members* instead of patients, and an expectation that some members at least may be actively involved in the club's activities.

The 'clubhouse' model[13] also fits in well with the growth of the 'user' movement in psychiatry and a philosophy which attempts to treat patients much more like ordinary people with problems, rather than as incapable, incompetent invalids who are not interested in contributing to their own care. Therapy can then be delivered in other, more appropriate, settings. Some of the best examples of these clubs are to be found in the work of local user groups, rather than in statutory sector provisions.

Drop-in support facilities offer alternative, relatively undemanding opportunities for social contact and support to those long-term patients who do not wish (or are not able) to be involved actively in their own care. They are often a feature of user-led clubs. However, it must be emphasised that a 'drop in' centre can seldom meet *all* patients' needs and there is a danger that the 'drop in' becomes a 'drop out'. Rest and relaxation should be a counterpoint to work and activity and it is therefore important—just as with residential provisions—to aim for an individually-centred 'package' of care which uses a range of work and social supports geared to different levels of need and different levels of functioning. Only in this way, can the full range of individual needs be met.

Mobile Staff Resources

Effective community care is about much more than simply an array of fixed facilities. It is also about providing flexible and mobile help which will take services to people in their own homes and provide variable levels of care tailored to suit individual needs. This will necessitate considerable changes in the disposition of personnel and in the pattern of service delivery.

This has particular implications for the role of staff like CPNs. Many GPs have become accustomed to CPNs who are 'outposted' to surgeries and work closely with the primary health care team. This model works well where the CPN is focusing on people with relatively specific problems and where a single, discrete intervention (e.g. a course of anxiety management or cognitive treatment for depression) may be all that is required.

However, for those with more severe and generalised problems—as in the case of schizophrenia—the CPN should be part of a specialist, multidisciplinary team. They need to be able to draw on other members of the team for specialist expertise (e.g. regarding medication, psychological approaches to coping with psychotic symptoms, family interventions, etc.) and they need to be working as part of a team so as to be able to preserve consistency and continuity of care. In the future, we may therefore expect to see the development of specialised multidisciplinary teams which will offer both treatment and management in the community, on an 'out of hours', as well as on a weekday basis. As yet, there are few examples in this country of such services[14], although there is increasing recognition of their value[15].

Experience in other countries (mainly the USA and Australia) suggests that such specialised community-based teams can significantly reduce numbers of admissions and lengths of stay in hospital without any disadvantages in terms of symptomatic recovery[16,17]. There also seems to be significant possible advantages in terms of social and domestic functioning, and both patients and their families consistently *prefer* community-based treatment, providing it is part of a comprehensive package of care. 'Crisis' services and mobile, intensive community support teams are therefore likely to be a much more prominent feature of community mental health services in the future and we may look forward to a time where such facilities are regarded as just as fundamental as inpatient beds and residential accommodation.

Case or care management

One final element which must be mentioned in the context of community supports is the idea of 'case' or 'care' management. **'Case management'** is a term which originated in the United States. The concept was invented in response to the perceived failure of community programmes to deal with the problems of the long-term mentally ill, particularly those with schizophrenia. The central idea is a simple one: people with complicated and long-term needs for services require a single point in the system (ie, an individual or a team) which will co-ordinate inputs, monitor progress, and maintain continuity over time. In the current context, it is intended that this will be delivered by two complementary initiatives—the *'Care Programme Approach'* (CPA) which is to be implemented by Health authorities and *'Care Management'* in which local Social Service departments are to take the lead role.

A description of the two approaches is to be found in a series of circulars from the Department of Health from 1990 onwards and is summarised in the guidance to the White Paper 'Caring for People'[18]. The essential distinction rests on the extent to which they include *'purchasing'*, as well as *'providing'* functions. Care programming essentially consists only of direct service provision and does not usually involve purchasing, whereas care 'management' has purchasing as its central task, together with a smaller element of direct service provision in terms of needs assessment, 'brokerage' (i.e. liaison with providers) and ongoing monitoring. The CPA was therefore designed to build on existing good practice by systematising procedures, clarifying responsibilities, and improving the continuity of care. Care management was meant to encourage Social Service departments to adopt a more flexible, 'needs-led, as opposed to 'service-led', approach. 'Packages' of care were to be constructed based on a careful assessment of individual's needs, rather than on the simple availability of standard service inputs.

Implementation of the CPA is still patchy and there is some confusion from having two rather similar approaches, aimed at similar objectives, being deployed in parallel by the two major statutory agencies[19]. There is also some evidence of the implementation of care management adversely affecting inter-agency working and leading to fragmentation of community teams[20]. This has led to calls for a rationalisation of the two procedures (including the arrangements for patients discharged under Section 117) into a single system which would combine *both* the direct service elements of the CPA and the purchasing element of care management[21]. Such a system would also make it much easier to implement the requirements of the new 'Supervision Registers' which relate to a subset of those who should already be cared for under the CPA.

Evidence on the effectiveness of case management systems suggests that they can be useful in maintaining patients in the community and improving social and occupational functioning. However, the results largely depend on the extent to which case managers are really prepared to be actively involved in 'outreach' work, and to be available on an 'out-of-hours' basis.

The research also highlights the importance of integrating care managers into the existing services and not expecting them to solve all the problems of inter and intra agency co-operation on their own[22]. There is thus a paradox in case management, in that it aims to solve the problems of co-ordination and continuity of care, but it cannot do so unless there are already good working relationships 'on the ground'.

The Cambridge Health District

An example of community services for the long-term mentally ill

Community provisions do vary a great deal in different parts of the country. Many inner city areas have specific local problems of poverty and social deprivation which make the development of good public services extremely difficult. Nevertheless, there are examples of good community care and these are not all confined to prosperous, middle class areas[23,24]. In order to illustrate some of the ideas, I will now draw on examples from the service in the Cambridge Health District.

The Cambridge Health District serves a population of approximately 270,000 people. It is a mixed rural/urban area with the main town (Cambridge city, population approx. 110,000) situated more or less in the middle of the catchment area. The district is relatively prosperous with low levels of social deprivation. Until recently, unemployment levels were also generally low. The local economy is dominated by the university and other educational institutions and there has been a recent growth in 'high tech' and service industries. Mental health services are centred around Fulbourn Hospital which is located about four miles from the town centre. There are acute, long-stay, and psychogeriatric beds on site, but outpatients are seen away from the mental hospital, at locations in the city or local health centres. The general psychiatric service is sectorised, with each sector looking after approximately 80,000 people. The hospital provides a base for 'outreach' into the network of day services and sheltered accommodation in the community (see below). An acute unit and outpatient services are to be developed on the general hospital site (Addenbrookes) situated about a mile down the road, but there are no plans to close Fulbourn itself. The rehabilitation and continuing care services, which deal with most of the people with chronic schizophrenia, have a good reputation and the district has been designated by the Department of Health a *National Demonstration Centre* for psychiatric rehabilitation.

In terms of residential provisions there are currently more than 180 places (approx 65 per 100,000) available in sheltered accommodation specifically for the mentally ill. These comprise 67 places (36%) in hostels providing 24–hour cover; 32 places (18%) in 'supported' group homes and 'bed-sits' with daily staff visiting; and 83 places (46%) in unstaffed accommodation (eg, group homes, flats). Most of these places (more than 80%) are provided by the independent sector, and one housing association (Granta Housing Society) provides over half the total. There have been considerable benefits to the health authority in working with a single housing agency in terms of developing a shared approach to care and a close working partnership, based on mutual respect, now exists.

In addition to this range of sheltered accommodation in the community, there are also 20 places for '*new*' long-stay patients in two ward-in-a-house developments (n=8 and 12) in the hospital. These cater for the most difficult of the younger patients who cannot be managed in the community. Nearly all have a diagnosis of schizophrenia. It is recognised that there is a need for more highly supervised, permanent accommodation and more mobile community support.

In terms of day care, there are about 120 places available each day in seven different centres, mainly based in the city. About half the places (3 centres) are essentially *work-orientated*, while the other half provide *social* and *therapeutic activities.* One of the work projects (Castle Project Workshop) is run by the Richmond Fellowship and provides high quality sheltered work in the form of furniture restoration, printing and toy manufacture. It sells its goods and services direct to the public, or through local shops and galleries and has recently set up a small, independent, co-operative business which aims to offer permanent employment—without subsidy—to six people with long-term mental illness. The Castle Project also runs a placement scheme, finding people part-time positions in local industry.

There is also a user-led social club (*Gemini*), funded by Social Services, operating in a building which it shares with the local public library. Fifteen to twenty people attend each day and there is space to 'drop-in', but the emphasis is on activity and sharing responsibility for running the club between the members and a small staff team. A 'clubhouse' is also being planned.

One of the other day centres (funded by the health authority) provides a base for a case management system with multidisciplinary staff team which offers comprehensive assessment of needs, co-ordination, and monitoring of progress for more than 150 long term patients living in the community[25]. In addition to these formal services, the local MIND group runs a 'befriending' scheme for over a hundred clients, and considerable use is made of a range of ordinary community facilities (eg, adult education classes, the Womens' Resources Centre, local church groups).

In terms of mobile staff resources, there are 6.5 whole-time CPNs working in the rehabilitation service, plus a full time community occupational therapist. These staff provide a seven-day service, but do not work 'out-of-hours'. There is also a separate 'community support team' consisting of a full-time psychologist, occupational therapist and part-time psychiatrist. The team visit the sheltered accommodation and provide back-up and training for staff, many of whom are not professionally trained. Unfortunately, this team can only cover weekdays and emergencies still have to be dealt with by the duty doctor system. There is no functioning crisis team in the district. This is clearly a need for the future.

Conclusion

The management of schizophrenia in the community is not easy. It is often said that care in the community may sound desirable in theory, but in practice it has failed to live up to expectations. There is some truth in this, and there are certainly considerable variations in services in different parts of the country. These variations reflect a host of specific local factors such as demography, population density, social deprivation and traditional attitudes which make it difficult to generalise about the 'success' or 'failure' of community care policies. Some degree of local variation is clearly inevitable. Indeed, it is desirable, since no 'blueprint' for planning services is universally applicable. However, the extent of variation which currently exists is too great. In order to ensure that there are minimum standards for the range and quality of provisions, there must be consensus of local professionals with shared ideas, vision and a will to get things done. GPs form a vital part of this consensus. Of course, ideas and determination will not be enough on their own, and resources will also have to be made available. But, if people have a clear view about what is needed, they can present a united front to those who have the responsibility to see that resources are allocated to meet these needs. Hopefully, the principles upon which services for people with schizophrenia should be based are now clear.

In the end it will be up to those 'on the ground' to see that these ideas are translated into reality.

References

1. World Health Organisation. *Schizophrenia: an international follow-up study* Chichester: Wiley, 1979
2. Warner, R. *Recovery from schizophrenia.* London: Routledge, 1985
3. Birchwood, M., Shepherd, G. Controversies and growing points in cognitive–behavioural interventions for people with schizophrenia. *Behavioural Psychotherapy* 1992;**20**:305–342.
4. Thornicroft, G., Breakey, W. The COSTAR programme. 1: Improving social networks of the long-term mentally ill. *British Journal of Psychiatry* 1991;**159**:245–249.
5. Garety, P.A. Housing. In: Lavender A., Holloway F., eds. *Community care in practice.* Chichester: Wiley, 1988;143–159.
6. Morris, I. Residential care. In: Bennett, D.H., Freeman, H.L., eds. *Community psychiatry..* London: Churchill Livingstone, 1991.
7. Wing, J.K. *Epidemiologically-Based Mental Health Needs Assessment.* London: Royal College of Psychiatrists Research Unit, 1992
8. Lavender, A. Quality of care and staff practices in long-stay settings. In: Watts, F.N., ed. *New developments in clinical psychology.* Chichester:Wiley, 1986.
9. Bennett, D.H., The chronic psychiatric patient today. J R Soc Med 1980; **73(4)** 301–303.
10. Young, R. *Residential Needs of Severely Disabled Psychiatric Patients—The Case for Hospital Hostels.* London: HMSO, 1991.
11. Shepherd, G., King, C., Fowler, D.G. Outcomes in Hospital Hostels. *Psychiatric Bulletin* 1994;**18**:619–612.
12. Pilling, S. Work and the continuing care client. In: Lavender, A., Holloway, F., eds. *Community care in practice.* Chichester: Wiley, 1988;187–205.
13. Beard, J., Propst, R.N., Malamud, T. J. The Fountain House Model of psychiatric rehabilitation. *Psychosocial Rehabilitation Journal* 1982; **5**:47–53.
14. Ford, R., Beadsmoore, A., Ryan, P., Repper, J., Craig, T., Muijen, M. Providing the safety net: Case management for people with serious mental illness. *Journal of Mental Health* 1995'**4**:91–97.
15. Audit Commission *Finding a Place.* London: HMSO, 1994.
16. Burns, B.J., Santos, A.B. (1995) Assertive Community Treatment: An Update of Randomised Trials. *Psychiatric Services* 1995;**46**:669–675.
17. Muijen, M., Marks, M., Connolly, B., Audini, B., McNamee, G. The Daily Living Programme. Preliminary comparison of community versus hospital based treatment for the seriously mentally ill facing emergency admission. *British Journal of Psychiatry* 1992;**160**:379–384.
18. Department of Health. *Caring for people: community care in the next decade and beyond: policy guidance.* London: HMSO, 1990. (cm.849).
19. Shepherd, G. Finding A Place: A review of mental health services for adults. *Journal of Mental Health* 1995;**4**:9–16.
20. Editorial—Care management: a disastrous mistake. *Lancet* 1995;**345**:399–401.
21. Mental Health Foundation *Creating Community Care: A Report of the Mental Health Foundation Inquiry into Community Care for People with Severe Mental Illness.* London:Mental Health Foundation, 1994.

[22] Shepherd, G. Case management. *Health Trends* 1990; **22**: 59–61.

[23] Lovett, A. A house for all seasons: the role of housing in community care. In: Reed, J., Lomas, G. eds. *Psychiatric services in the communty.* London: Croom Helm, 1984 91–100.

[24] Howat, J., Bates, P., Pidgeon J., Shepperson, G. The development of residential accomodation in the community. In: Lavender, A., Holloway, F. , eds. *Community care in practice.* Chicester: Wiley, 1988; 275–293.

[25] Shepherd, G., Tilbury, J., King, C., Fowler, D. Implementing the Care Programme Approach. *Journal of Mental Health* 1995; **4:**261–274.

Further reading

Watts, F. N., Bennett, D.H., eds. *Theory and practice of psychiatric rehabilitation.* Chichester: Wiley, 1991.

Weller, M., Muijen, M. eds. *Dimensions of Community Care,* London: Saunders, 1994.

Address for Contact

Professor Geoff Shepherd, Head of Research, The Sainsbury Centre for Mental Health, 134–138 Borough High Street, London, SE1 1LB

6 Schizophrenia: Early Detection, Early Intervention

PETER TYRER, Professor of Community Psychiatry, St Charles Hospital, London

SUMMARY

The view that early detection of schizophrenia leading to intervention and appropriate treatment is likely to be beneficial seems to make sense. Unfortunately it has not been demonstrated in practice partly because early detection is often hampered by bureaucratic referral systems and by the tendency for schizophrenia to present late in its course. The work of the Early Intervention Service, a community-based mental health team in central London, is described. Because it operates an open referral system and assesses patients within days early intervention and treatment is achieved. The results from a recently completed controlled trial of patients presenting as emergencies and randomly allocated to the Early Intervention Service or the standard hospital service showed greater symptomatic improvement, service satisfaction, and a significant reduction in days admitted to hospital (most marked for patients with schizophrenia) in those allocated to early intervention. Mainly because of an 8–fold reduction in bed days the costs incurred by the patients treated by early intervention were 40 per cent of those incurred by the standard group. There is scope for similar services being introduced elsewhere but appropriate training and resources are required which would cost the health service more in the short-term before the gains are realised.

Introduction

This subject matches a strategy of treatment *(early intervention)* with a serious psychiatric disorder *(schizophrenia)*. Despite the obvious face validity of the equation:

Early Detection + Early Intervention = Early Cure

there is no real evidence that this formula is true in the case of schizophrenia. In understanding why there is such an important gap in our knowledge, it is important to appreciate that early intervention originates from a different standpoint than the treatment of schizophrenia.

Crisis intervention

The principle of crisis intervention was formulated primarily by the work of Caplan in 1964[1]. The implications lying behind such intervention was that the population being treated was essentially normal; had been placed under a combination of stresses that led to a crisis (almost invariably an emotional crisis); and was associated with breakdown of functioning and relationships.

Expressed mechanistically, a crisis is the upset of a steady state[2]. Caplan viewed this period as far more than an emotional problem needing support and solution. He regarded a crisis as "a transition period presenting an individual with an opportunity of personality growth and with the danger of increased vulnerability to mental disorder, the outcome of which in any particular instant, to some extent depends on his way of handling the situation, and is to be contrasted with earlier views of stress or trauma as aetiological factors in mental disorder[1]. One of the main aims of crisis intervention is to maximise these opportunities for growth as well as to avoid mental disorder developing.

Crisis intervention is a short-term therapy which is brought to operation as early as possible, so that the best assessment can be made and because people in crisis are more receptive to change. Successful crisis intervention involves the return to a steady state in which there is emotional adjustment again and, sometimes as a bonus, confers additional resources to the person by promoting what is perceived as personality growth.

Schizophrenia

Although there have been many views about the aetiology of schizophrenia since it was first described by Bleuler[3], there is now little argument that it is best viewed as a disease, involving at least *two sub-groups*: (i) an acute group with many positive symptoms; and (ii) a more chronic group characterised by negative features[4]. Schizophrenia can achieve a steady state, but this is not a normal state and the notion of crisis intervention in the short-term to restore health to an essentially normal individual can hardly apply to schizophrenia. The time course of intervention is also different in schizophrenia from neurotic and adjustment disorders. In order to be confident that an intervention has been effective, one needs a long period of follow up, to establish that the disorder has not recurred. To date there have been no appropriate studies of such primary intervention, although in Buckinghamshire, Ian Falloon is currently looking at this type of intervention after the success of home-based therapy (based on behavioural treatment) as practised on the west coast of America[5].

Most of the interest in different types of intervention in schizophrenia has revolved round the alternatives of hospital and community treatment[6] and the value of social intervention to limit the extent and the impact of "high expressed emotion"[7] (see chapter one). However, these approaches can be regarded as forms of secondary or tertiary prevention. By the time they are instituted the diagnosis of schizophrenia has been well established and the efficacy of the intervention is best determined by the frequency of relapse.

The Early Intervention Service

The absence of adequate data demonstrating the adequacy of early intervention, does not mean that services orientated towards early identification and treatment should concentrate only on non-psychotic disorders. The *Early Intervention Service* (EIS) is a community mental health team working in the Paddington and North Kensington area of Inner London (the southern half of Parkside District Health Authority). This team has 10 members: one psychiatrist (the author), a psychologist, three community mental health nurses, two social workers, two occupational therapists, and an administrator. It serves a population of approximately 120,000 packed into a densely-populated area of four square miles.

This area faces particular problems, having a large number of different ethnic groups, a gross shortage of adequate primary care facilities (30 per cent of the population do not have a GP), and major housing problems—including a large proportion of residents placed in bed-and-breakfast accommodation from other London boroughs. The EIS is primarily concerned with major psychiatric disorder, so it is not surprising that a large proportion of referrals suffer from schizophrenia and associated conditions. Diagnosis of all patients seen is made using the new ICD–10 classification[8] and nearly a quarter (23.5 per cent) of all patients seen have a diagnosis of schizophrenia or an associated disorder using this system[9].

Because of the problems in providing comprehensive medical cover for this population, the EIS accepts referrals from all sources and although GPs represent the largest single referral group (35 per cent), 20 other groups refer also. The aim of this service is to see patients as soon as possible after referral, in the most appropriate setting. For half the patients, that is at home.

The EIS does not offer a 24–hour cover so cannot be regarded strictly as a crisis intervention service such as that operating in the London Borough of Barnet[10] and other authorities. Nevertheless, it can respond quickly to referrals, and only very few patients are not engaged. The service is also successful in engaging patients referred as emergencies to the psychiatric services. A formal comparison has recently been completed of patients presenting as psychiatric emergencies to St Mary's Hospital, Paddington. Patients deemed to be in need of psychiatric treatment were randomly allocated to the EIS or to the standard hospital service and assessed by independent investigators masked to knowledge of service received over the next 12 weeks[11]. In addition to assessments of diagnosis and symptom severity, patients also had their social functioning and networks recorded, and at the end of 12 weeks their satisfaction with the service received was measured using a questionnaire. A separate record of all medical, psychiatric and related services received was also made.

Types of intervention in schizophrenia

Data from this formal comparison are still being collected. However, it is useful to examine differences which exist between the EIS approach and the more typical psychiatric services with regard to the presentation and management of schizophrenia (Table 6.1).

There are roughly equal referrals made by medical agencies (general practitioners 35 per cent, other doctors 13 per cent) and non-medical ones (52 per cent). Non-medical referrals include social workers (20 per cent), self-referrals (7 per cent), health visitors (6 per cent), residential agencies (including hostels) (3 per cent) and over 15 other agencies. An investigation of the types of referral revealed the important finding that general practitioners and other doctors referred significantly fewer cases of severe mental illness to the service than the non-medical ones[12]. Although this may be a reflection of the particular problems experienced by psychiatric services in central London it indicates the advantages of an open referral system in such areas. In fact, we find that one of the least skilled referrers, in terms of professional or psychiatric knowledge (housing agencies), refers the most disturbed patients. Referrals are usually presented to the EIS before admission is considered to be essential. Because the service is community-orientated, if the problems presented by the patient are so great that the referrer believes there is no alternative to admission, then the appropriate service is sought—usually via the local hospital's accident and emergency department.

Table 6.1: *Comparison between community intervention (Early Intervention Service) and more typical services for schizophrenia, London 1990*

	Early Intervention Service (EIS)	Typical psychiatric service
Referral	More frequently from non-medical agencies	Almost all from medical agencies
Presentation	Usually before admission considered essential	Often at time when admission is felt to be mandatory
Place of assessment	Usually at home or non-medical setting	Usually hospital or outpatient setting
Type of treatment	Drug and family treatment together with close liaison with other agencies	Primary drug therapy in a medical setting

The place of assessment often differs, and although exceptions occur[13], it is still relatively rare nowadays for schizophrenic patients to be seen at home for their first assessment, particularly in inner cities. The EIS is unusual in this respect, although it is appreciated that home assessments are undoubtedly more expensive than hospital ones.

The type of treatment given is also a little different in the community service, although there is no fundamental difference of philosophy. In a typical psychiatric service there is a danger that the management of schizophrenia becomes drug treatment only, and the response to this is all-important in the continued progress of the patient. All organisations involved in the community treatment of schizophrenia are aware of the importance of family treatment (which, in our area, has to be extended to include people with whom the person is living, as relatively few patients are living with their families).

Although the work of the EIS does not include formal programmes to improve behaviour and reduce high expressed emotions (such as those discussed by Professor Leff in chapter one), it does adopt the same general strategies. One of the major problems of the newer treatments is that they are difficult to carry out away from major research centres because of the number of staff required. It would certainly be helpful to have cheaper versions of these approaches which were less labour-intensive, but still effective.

Close liaison with other agencies is an important part of the work of the EIS and in the Central London area where we work, the major contact is with housing. It is often paradoxically more difficult to get appropriate housing for the patients when they are treated in the community, because the pressure to be rehoused is often stronger when the patient is occupying a hospital bed unnecessarily.

Figure 6.1: *Mean numbers of inpatient bed days occupied by patients after random allocation to the Early Intervention Service (EIS) and standard hospital service(S) over a 12–week period, separated by diagnostic status using the ICD–10 classification*

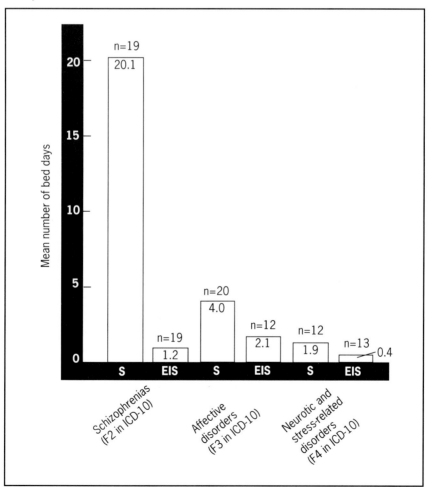

*Four patients with alcohol-related diagnosis (F1 in ICD–10) are not included as none of these had inpatient care during the 12 weeks.

Because the EIS and other teams which have an approach linked to crisis intervention do not see patients over a long period, the importance of the GP maintaining treatment and contact cannot be overstated. If it can be shown that early intervention in an individual case can prevent admission and maintain treatment in a primary care setting, this will be used as a blue-print for the future to avoid the *damaging cycle* of *admission, discharge* and *readmission*, so common in psychiatric practice. This can be made effective only by creating good relationships between the community psychiatric service, the patient (and/or family) and the GP. Close liaison between all three is essential. There is certainly reason to believe that if the patient presents for treatment as soon as symptoms re-emerge (and before insight is lost), successful treatment can be implemented. This will then prevent the patient from following the *common path of isolation, personal disruption and compulsory admission*.

Results of trial of early intervention in schizophrenia

Of 100 patients included in the study, 38 had a diagnosis in the schizophrenia group (using ICD–10 criteria with consensus diagnosis achieved by a panel). Nineteen each were allocated to the EIS and the standard service. For the group taken as a whole, there was significantly greater improvement in symptoms in patients allocated to the EIS compared to the standard service, but no difference in social function or social networks. Patients were also significantly more satisfied with the EIS than the standard service[11].

Separate analyses showed patients with schizophrenia were similar to those with other diagnoses with regard to all these variables. During the 12–week period of the study, most patients in both services were treated as outpatients but, despite this, significantly greater numbers of days in hospital (bed days) were used by the standard service. Analysis by diagnosis showed that by far the largest part of the difference was accounted for by patients with schizophrenia (F-ratio (interaction between diagnosis and service group) 4.2; df 2.89; $p < 0.02$) (see Figure 6.1).

Examinations of costs showed that, although the median cost of treatment was higher in the patients treated by the EIS (£938) compared with the standard group (£610), this disguised the large costs incurred by the minority of in-patients treated. The total cost of treatment of the EIS-treated patients was £56,000, 43 per cent of the sum incurred by the patients in the standard group[14], which illustrates some of the difficulties that are involved in cost-benefit analysis.

The time scale employed in this study was a short one and we have no evidence that the benefits of early intervention are maintained over a longer period. Nevertheless, these findings are encouraging. They reinforce evidence from other studies that community intervention reduces the need for hospital care[6,12,15] and may confer additional benefits of possible long-term significance.

Conclusions

Early intervention in schizophrenia is not an easy option, because patients with this condition are less easy to engage than those with most psychiatric disorders. Nevertheless, the findings from the EIS and other community psychiatric initiatives suggest that there are systems of care which offer better alternatives to standard approaches to treatment. The treatment involves no dramatic breakthroughs, but merely allows the service to reach the patient at an appropriate time and setting so that disruption is minimised and treatment is more likely to be a collaborative than a confrontational exercise.

Acknowledgements

I thank my colleges at the Early Intervention Service and Drs Sarah Marriott and Stephen Merson for their advice over the content of this paper, Jonathan Tyrer and Tony Johnson for statistical help, and the World Health Organisation for permission to use and quote from the draft versions of the tenth revision of Chapter V of the International Classification of Diseases.

References

[1] Caplan, G. *Principles of preventative psychiatry.* New York: Basic Books, 1964.

[2] Parad, H. The use of time-limited crisis intervention in community mental health programming. *Social Service Review* 1966: **40**: 275–282.

[3] Bleuler, E. *Dementia praecox or the group of schizophrenia.* 1911: (translated by Zinkin JJ). New York: International Universities Press, 1950.

[4] Crow, T.J. Molecular pathology of schizophrenia: more than one disease process? *BMJ* 1980: **280**: 66–68.

[5] Falloon, I.R.H., Boyd, J.L., McGill, C.W. et al. Family management in the prevention of morbidity in schizophrenia. *Archives of General Psychiatry* 1985; **42**: 887–896.

[6] Hoult, J., Reynolds, I. Schizophrenia: a comparative trial of community-oriented and hospital-oriented psychiatric care. *Acta Psychiatrica Scandinavica* 1985; **69**: 359–372.

[7] Leff, J., Kuipers, L., Berkowitz, R., Eberlein-Vries, R., Sturgeon, D. A. controlled trial of social intervention in the families of schizophrenic patients. *British Journal of Psychiatry* 1982; **141**: 121–134.

[8] World Health Organisation. *International Classification of Diseases: draft 10th revision.* Geneva: WHO, 1988.

[9] Onyett, S. Liaison between Primary and Secondary Care Teams Towards Early Intervention: Assertive Help for Inner City Distress, In R. Jenkins, J. Newton and R. Young (Eds), *The Prevention of Depression and Anxiety in General Practice—the role of the primary care team.* London: HMSO, 1992.

[10] Scott, R.D. A family oriented psychiatric service to the London Borough of Barnet. *Health Trends* 1980; **3**: 65–68.

[11] Merson, S., Tyrer, P., Onyett, S., Lynch, S., Lack, S. A controlled evaluation of early intervention in psychiatric emergencies. *Lancet* 1992; **339**: 1311–14

[12] Marriott, S., Malone, S., Onyett, S., Tyrer, P. The consequences of an open referral system to a community mental health service. *Acta Psychiatrica Scandinavica* 1993; **88**: 93–97.

[13] Jones, S.J., Turner, R.J., Grant, J.E. Assessing patients in their homes. *Bulletin of Royal College of Psychiatrists* 1987; **11**: 117–119.

[14] Merson, S., Tyrer, P., Carlen, D. and Johnson, A.L. (1995). The cost of treatment of psychiatric emergencies: a comparison of hospital and community services. *Psychological Medicine*, (in press).

[15] Tyrer, P. and Creed, F. (eds). *Community psychiatry in action.* Cambridge: Cambridge University Press, 1995.

7 The Interface Between Community Mental Health Teams and Primary Care in the Management of Individuals with Schizophrenia

GERALDINE STRATHDEE, Consultant Psychiatrist, PACT team, The Bethlem and Maudsley NHS Trust, London.

SUMMARY

The role of the general practitioner in caring for those with long-term mental health disorders has been ignored to a large extent. The community care movement, with its dual emphasis on reducing the number of long-stay hospital beds and treating patients in their homes has resulted in more patients with severe and chronic illness moving into communities. Research demonstrates that for many patients the general practitioner may be, not only the first point of contact in crisis, but also the only provider of professional health care. It is therefore vital that the development of community psychiatric services include organisational structures which facilitate liaison and communication with GPs. General practitioners in turn, need to reassess and clarify their own role and education in dealing with this client group.

This paper describes the development of two community psychiatric services which attempted, from inception, to liaise and integrate with their sector general practitioners. In no sense comprehensive, it presents some organisational structures evolved to facilitate the liaison; details the role of the GP in the care of people with schizophrenia formulated by discussion between the community mental health and primary care teams, the users, carers and other community agencies; expands on ways in which care can be improved for individuals with schizophrenia through the development of practice case registers and policies and the involvement of primary care professionals in the Care Programme Approach.

Primary care and the seriously mentally ill

The seminal work of Shepherd et al[1] and Goldberg & Bridges[2] demonstrated that between one–fifth and one–quarter of patients present a psychological problem as either their sole or major difficulty to their GP. Just over half of them have chronic disorders, defined as continually present for at least a year, or recurring with sufficient frequency to cause continuous disability or require prophylactic treatment. Similar figures have been found in other countries. For example, in the US Regier *et al.*[3] demonstrated that over thirty per cent of primary care patients had a diagnosis of mental disorder, and of these, nine percent suffered chronic disability.

Table 7.1 illustrates the average GP's workload in respect of patients with mental disorders[4].

Table 7.1 *Mental health conditions in primary care*

Diagnosis	Rates per 1000 population per year	Number of patients in a practice of 2010 per year
Schizophrenia	2–6	4–12
Affective psychosis	3.0	6–7
Organic dementia	2.2	4–5
Depression	30–50	60–100
Anxiety and other neuroses	35.7	70–80
Situational disturbances/other diagnoses	26.7	50–60
Drug/alcohol disorder	2.7	5–6

The number of individuals with schizophrenia is increased where the practice is located near a closing long-stay psychiatric hospital, in urban areas and where the GP has had an interest or specialist training in psychiatry. Individual GPs have relatively few patients with schizophrenia on their lists, but, without the provision of high quality, effective care, these patients can consume a disproportionate amount of practice time and energy.

In psychiatric circles there is a frequently held belief that the all the seriously mentally ill are cared for by the secondary services and that primary care is exclusively the province of the 'walking well'. This claim can be refuted by the considerable body of evidence which has accrued and which substantiates the central role of the primary care team.

In 1962, Murray-Parkes[5] followed up a cohort of patients with schizophrenia discharged from London mental hospitals. He found that over 70 per cent had seen their GP in the year after discharge, half of them having consulted *more than* five times. In the same period, less than three-fifths had attended hospital outpatient departments, and of these most had been seen *less than* five times. Johnstone[6] in 1984, studying a similar group of discharged patients found that just under a quarter (24%) were seeing **only** their GP. In a review of all those with schizophrenia in the Camden area who had once been in contact with the service, Pantelis *et al.*[7] found that only 60 per cent still retained contact. However, when community mental health services are more developed and integrated with primary care, those who traditionally drop out of secondary care ie. young, male, paranoid men and older women with schizophrenia are more likely to attend for specialist care[8].

Table 7.2 develops, from the primary care viewpoint, a model of the effects of de-institutionalisation. It seems inevitable that the continuing trend towards community care in psychiatry will result in increasing clinical, educative and supportive demands being placed on GPs and other members of the primary health care team. Therefore there is a need for community mental health teams to work in an integrated and effective manner with them.

Table 7.2 *THE IMPACT OF COMMUNITY CARE ON THE GP WORKLOAD*

Community Care Strategy	Impact on GPs
Closure of large psychiatric hospitals	Greater number of patients with long-term disorders on list More group homes and hostels on list
Less available hospital beds	More patients treated at home and in the community Less access to respite facilities
Shorter length of stay	More acute illness treated at home Increased intervention with psychotropic medication
First point of contact for the severely ill	Increased crisis intervention Increased Mental Health Act use
New ways of working	Need to understand and participate in the Care Programme Approach
New effective treatment techniques	Use of psychoeducational approaches Development of crisis contracts Help with relapse prevention techniques Use of problem solving techniques with families Use of case register and guidelines (as used in diabetes and asthma) Support role for families and carers.

A sectorised community psychiatric service

My previous paper in this series[9] outlined a range of practical interventions which can help GPs assess and manage patients with both minor and severe mental disorders. This article focuses on strategies relevant to the latter group and describes in some detail the organisation of two services which facilitated their implementation. It is written from the perspective of community populations of between 40–45, 000, in the Greenwich and Southwark areas of South London.

The Greenwich Sector

The primary care infra-structure of the sector in Greenwich was organisationally ideal for liaison with a community mental health service. It was co-terminous with a Social Services area, and the majority of patients were served by GPs who worked from two large health centres and a group practice, were interested in psychiatry and already had sophisticated case registers and computerised records. A Social Services day centre, several group homes, and other sheltered housing facilities also operated there. The psychiatric team comprised a consultant psychiatrist, a senior house officer, a half-time psychologist, a community occupational therapist, four community psychiatric nurses: two were generic; one was a member of a specialist team who treated only the long-term mentally ill; and one formed a part of a community alcohol team. The team base and information system were located in a community mental health centre on the site of one of the local primary care health centres. Only the acute admission facilities were located outside the sector – at the district general hospital. Patients with severe, long-term mental health disorders received priority attention, and a fundamental objective of the developing community services was liaison and integration with the primary care services.

Service organisation in relation to primary care

Five organisational strategies were used:

First: A hospital outpatient clinic was replaced with a regular session in the largest health centre which cared for one–third of the sector patients. The aim was to develop a similar service with the second health centre. Both new referrals and follow-up patients were seen at the 'clinic', and face-to face discussions with the GPs enabled joint working with many patients.

Second: An additional clinic was replaced with a peripatetic system of *care-coordination clinics* at the local day centre and area social services office. These were the precursor of Care Programme Approach meetings.

Third: Two of the community psychiatric nurses and the community occupational therapist held regular sessions in the health centres. These included group sessions as an effective use of time and a way of helping with the significant workload.

Fourth: The most 'psychologically-minded' GP in the nearest practice involved with patients in each group home in the sector was identified. He or she was then contacted and efforts made to improve communication and professional support.

Fifth: A series of joint audit meetings was held between the sector team and GPs to discuss aspects of service delivery – eg, crisis intervention, the development of treatment, and good practice proformas.

The role of general practitioners in the care of individuals with schizophrenia

Tables 7.3 and 7.4 represent the results of many discussions held between the local GPs and members of the psychiatric team, and are an attempt to summarise the role of the GP at each stage of the illness.*

Table 7.3: *The role of the PHCT in the care of patients with schizophrenia*

New Presentations

> Detection and Identification
> Mental state Assessment
> Family Assessment
> Appropriate Referral
> User and Carer education
> Carer/Family support.

Continuing Care

> Assessment and treatment of physical morbidity
> Prescription and administration of medication
> Education of patients and carers
> Development of a trusting relationship
> Identification of patterns of relapse
> Monitoring the mental state
> Prevention of relapse
> Crisis Intervention
> Application of the Mental Health Act
> Liaison role with secondary care agencies
> Identification of local networks and supports
> Practical Advocacy
> Involvement in the Care Programme Approach.

Group Homes and Hostels

> Medical co-ordination
> Education and advice on psychotropic drugs
> Support role to carers.

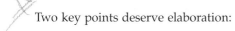

Two key points deserve elaboration:

(i) Initial identification and assessment

In Great Britain, GPs are often the first professionals contacted at the onset of a schizophrenic illness (see also page EDIT). As one senior GP said, 'It is only when I have known the family for a long time that I can detect the qualitative difference between a difficult adolescent who withdraws to his room and plays his stereo at maximum volume, and one who is at the pre-morbid stage of the development of a psychotic illness'.

The Present State Examination (PSE)[10] developed by the MRC Social Psychiatry Unit at the Maudsley Hospital, consists of a series of questions which fully

* Particular thanks are given to Drs. Ann Holden and Peter Lewins.

covers the range of experiences encountered by those with psychotic illnesses. I am not suggesting that the PSE be used in full, in a busy GP surgery! However, a brief re-read of the questionnaire can serve as an effective reminder of how best to conduct a mental state examination. Table 4 provides a useful checklist of items to cover when interviewing a patient with schizophrenia in the surgery or outpatient clinic.

Table 7.4: *A checklist for the consultation with a patient*

1.	Assessment of physical status.
2.	Advice on need for dental/chiropody/sight assessment.
3.	Mental state assessment (concurrent depression).
4.	Assessment of effect of medication.
5.	Medication history and administration.
6.	Evidence of tardive dyskinesia.
7.	Assessment of patient education level about their condition and treatment.
8.	Assessment of pre-morbid symptoms of relapse and prevention plan.
9.	Family/carer attitudes/education.
10.	Assessment of degree of social disability.
11.	Practical aids eg. bus pass.
12.	Assessment of need for social intervention.
13.	Assessment of skills and strengths.
14.	Clarification of relationship with secondary services.
15.	Written long-term management plans from the secondary services.

Fig 7.1: *The range of needs of individuals with mental health disorders*

NEEDS	The long-term mentally ill	Neurosis
Case-identification & case register recall	+++	+
Crisis intervention in the community & at home	+++	+
Medication	+++	+
Respite and crisis community beds	+++	+
Family education & support	+++	++
Maritial/sexual counselling	+	+++
Behavioural/cognitive therapies	+	+++
Supportive counselling	++	+++
Case management and assertive outreach	+++	+
Physical care	+++	+++
Social skills and stress management	+++	+++
Day care	+++	+
Welfare benefits advice	++	++
Housing	++	++
Legal advice	+	+
Support group/self-help group	++	+++
Information & education about illness and services	+++	+++

It is considered good practice to refer patients suspected of having schizophrenia **early** to a psychiatrist. However, every study on communication pattern between psychiatrists and GPs suggests that vital information is frequently omitted. Effective communication is extremely important, because, as Julian Leff discusses (see chapter 1), there is a strong interaction between the quality of the patient's environment and their prognosis. While the community mental health team may take several meetings to become familiar with the complex dynamics in the family situation, GPs are often only too aware of the tensions and stresses present. Unfortunately, perhaps awed by the jargon, they often fail to communicate these at referral or subsequently.

This can therefore lead to vital information being omitted. In order to improve the written communications between the teams a literature review of the relevant research was undertaken [11,12]. Table 5 summarises best practice

7.5

Table 7.5

What mental health professionals want in referral letters from the GP

- background family and social history
- details of presenting problems
- details of previous interventions and their effects
- current interventions, particularly current medication
- the reason for referral
- the service for the GP expects the psychiatrist to provide
- the GP's view of their continuing or transferred responsibilities.

What GPs want in communications from the community mental health team

- a clear management plan with an indication of treatment timescales, effects and possible side-effects, and the expected outcome
- indication of suicide risk
- what the patient has been told about their condition
- the prognosis and likely continuing disabilities and influence on the patient's life style
- the role of the GP and primary care team is expected to play in the management plan and the role to be played by the specialist staff
- indication of prescribing roles and responsibilities.

(ii) The continuing care role

The nature of the family doctor's role in providing continuing care to the patient will depend on the course and outcome of the illness. About a quarter of the patients recover completely; two–thirds continue to have occasional relapses (with mild to moderate degrees of social and functional impairment); and a tenth become severely disabled from an early stage [13].

The Nunhead sector

This section describes the strategies which have been used to develop close working practices with primary care teams in the second sector: a deprived inner city area of South London: the Nunhead area. Although the mental health team had a similar population size to the Greenwich sector the primary care infrastructure was very different. Instead of dealing with a core 3 to 4 practices, patients with mental health disorders were referred from a total of 26 practices and 47 GPs. The core practices in the patch were two large fund-holding practices, 5 larger (4 or more partner) group practices, the remainder being comprised of single handed GPs or small numbers of partners. This significantly 'challenged' the community teams to find methods of working closely with their primary counterparts. They developed a system which included:

First: A directory of all statutory and voluntary sector mental health services in the area was produced and sent to all sector GPs. This listed the organisations in the area undertaking treatment of the mentally ill. The contact name, address and telephone number of the organisation, the treatment provided, the likely effects of such treatment and number of sessions available was listed. The purpose was to assist the GPs in making appropriate referrals.

Second: Joint case-registers of the long-term mentally ill in the practices were set up. Table 7.6 indicates the sources of information for identifying the severely mentally ill. Table 7.7 lists the information agreed by the GPs and CHMTs as being the most important in assisting decision making.

Table 7.6: *What mental health professionals want in referral letters from the GP*

Primary Care Sources

- Recorded diagnosis of schizophrenia, manic-depression, other psychosis
- Repeat psychotropic drug prescriptions
- Frequent consultations for emergencies/home visits
- Depot injection administered
- CPN attenders
- Hostel/group home/sheltered residence populations
- Domiciliary visit requests
- Review of appointment/visit lists.

Local Mental Health Service Sources

- Case register of the long-term mentally ill
- Care Programme Approach register
- Outpatient attenders
- CPN case-loads
- Depot clinic patients
- Patients admitted under a section of the Mental Health Act
- Crisis attenders eg. A & E attenders
- Frequent in-patient admissions
- Residents of long-stay institutions
- Hostel/group home/sheltered residence populations.

Table 7.7: *Useful information to be recorded on the case-register?*

Socio-demographic data	name address tel no. age/sex marital status/household composition housing type no. children next of kin/carer address: tel no.
Clinical data	Diagnosis Suicide risk Indicators of relapse Specific crisis response Medication.
Service contact data	GP Psychiatrist CPN/case manager Needs assessment date Needs/problems identified and holistic care plan involved agency 1: tel no. involved agency 2: tel no. involved agency 3: tel no.
Practice Policy Recall	Last medication review Date physical review Next assessment date.

Third: Good practice protocols were developed at the request of local GPs. These were written using an interactive approach with the GPs. Titles include A general practitioner's Guide to: the Mental Health Act, Crisis Intervention, Good practice in the care of Individuals with Long-term Mental Health Disorders, Eating Disorders[15].

Fourth: Each practice had an identified link or liaison person to facilitate rapid transfer on information between the two teams.

Fifth: Bids were developed and put forward to the local FHSA on a locality commissioning model to obtain sessional attachments of dedicated primary care counsellors, psychologists and mental health nurses. The two localities comprised a number of geographically proximate practices. One was a cluster of two fund-holding practices, one large and the other small. The second grouping was of three non-fundholding practices, each with two to three partners. The aim was to give equity of access to specialist input to all practices. The staff were employed and managed by the CHMT's trust and monitored jointly by the GPs and community staff.

Sixth: Six monthly review meetings for patients on the Care Programme Approach were held with the larger practices. These took the form of a tightly managed one to two hour review of the care plans of all mutual mental health patients.

The Care Programme Approach

Individuals with schizophrenia have complex, multi-faceted needs and require a wide range of physical, psychological, social and other interventions (Fig 1). It is internationally accepted that the development of comprehensive community psychiatric services can only be achieved by a system which effectively co-ordinates all these aspects of care. The concept of case management has been found to achieve the best results. This is extensively used in modern psychiatric practice and incorporated into national policy by the introduction of the Care Programme Approach[13]. This aims to ensure that, for the most severely disabled patients, one individual or organisation takes the responsibility to assess and facilitate the provision of their needs in all the areas delineated during the assessment process.

Fundamental to the Care Programme Approach is the assessment of the health and social needs of patients by specialist mental health and social services. On the basis of this a care plan should be agreed with the patient. One person — a key worker — should be appointed and form the focal point of contact for the patient, carer, other staff members and primary health care team. This person is responsible for coordinating the delivery of mental and physical health and social care. He or she will also see that regular review and monitoring of the patient's needs and progress occurs.

What does this mean for the primary care professional?

The specialist psychiatric services should:

- invite a member of the PHCT to care planning and review meetings to assist in the formation of the care plan:

- through the keyworker find out the views and represent them if a member of the PHCT is unable to attend such meetings;

- give or send a copy of the care plan arising from a care plan or review meeting;

- inform the PHCT of the identity of the patient's key worker who should be in regular touch,

- inform the GP of emergency and out of hours contact numbers and plans.

The Primary Health Care Team should:

- always inform the specialist services of relevant changes in the patient's condition which may include the frequency and reasons for consultation, expressions of suicidal intent, effects of, or changes to, medication or other treatments;

- feed in information about the patient for care planning purposes, even if unable to attend the meeting itself;

- know how to get hold of the specialist services in a crisis as many severely mentally ill people will seek help from their GP first.

CMHTs nationally have developed several strategies to involve busy PHCTs in CPA meetings. These include: holding the CPA meeting in the GP surgery, arranging the meeting at a time convenient to the PHCT eg. after morning surgery or home visits, having regular six monthly reviews of all mutual clients to update information on the practice register.

Conclusion

Models which integrate primary and secondary care have the following benefits; reduction of hospital admissions and length of stay, earlier detection of psychiatric illness, a greater ability to promote relapse prevention, provision of care for those who are poor attenders at hospital clinics, increased patient and carer satisfaction.

As Professor Kathleen Jones[15], in her review of psychiatric services for the city of York concluded, that unless 'attention is given to finding administrative solutions to the repeated official exhortations for collaboration and co-operation with GPs we will fail to provide the mix of services needed'.

References

1. Shepherd, M., Cooper, B., Brown, A. & Kalton, G. *Psychiatric illness in general practice*. Oxford University Press 1966.
2. Goldberg, D. & Bridges, K. 'Screening for psychiatric illness in general practice: the general practitioner versus the screening questionnaire. *J R Coll Gen Practitioners* 1987; **37**: 15 –18.
3. Regier, D.A., Burke, J.R., Manderschied, R.W. & Burns, B.J. The chronically mentally ill in primary care. *Psycho Med* 1985; **15**: 265–273.
4. Strathdee, G. & Sutherby, K. Liaison psychiatry and primary health care settings. In *Multiprofessional Co-operation in Community mental Health Care*. Edward Arnold Publishers. 1995
5. Murray Parkes, C., Brown, G.W. & Monck, E. M. The general practitioner and the schizophrenic patient. *Br Med J* 1962; **1**: 972–6.
6. Johnstone, E., Owens, D., Gold, A., Crow, T. & MacMillan, J. Schizophrenic patients discharged from hospital — a follow-up study. *Br J Psych* 1964; **145**: 586–590.
7. Pantelis, C., Taylor, J. & Campbell, P. The South Camden schizophrenia survey. *Bull R Coll Psychiatrists* 1988; **12**: 89–101.
8. Brown, G., Strathdee, G., Christie-Brown, J.C.B. & Robinson, P.H. A comparison of referrals to primary care and hospital outpatient clinics. *Br J Psych* 1988; **153**: 168–173.
9. Strathdee, G. Liaison between primary and secondary care teams towards early intervention. *In Prevention of Depression and Anxiety in General Practice*. Jenkins, R., Newton, J. & Young, R. 1991.

[10] Wing, J.K. *Measurement and Classification of Psychiatric Symptoms*. Oxford University Press 1974.

[11] Williams, P. & Wallace, B. General Practitioners and Psychiatrists —Do They Communicate? British Medical Journal 1974; **1**: 505–507.

[12] Pullen, I.M. & Yellowlees, A. Is communication improving between general practitioners and psychiatrists? British Medical Journal 1985; **153**: 663–666.

[13] Englehart, D., Rosen, B., Feldman, J., Englehart, J. & Cohen, P. A 15 year follow-up study of 646 schizophrenic outpatients. *Sch Bull* 1982; **8**: 493—503.

[14] Strathdee, G. & Phelan, M. (eds) Maudsley Practical Clinical Handbook Series. Editions include:

Phelan, M., Strathdee, G. & Holden, A. (1993) A General Practitioner's Guide to the Mental Health Act. No. 1. *London: Boots Pharmaceuticals.*

Myers, S., Davies, M.P. & Treasure, J. (1993) A General Practitioner's Guide to Eating Disorders. No.2. *London: Boots Pharmaceuticals.*

Phelan, M., Hobson, A., & Hunter, R. (1993) A General Practitioner's Guide to Crisis Intervention. No.3. *London: Boots Pharmaceuticals.*

Strathdee, G. & Kendrick, T. (1995) A General Practitioner's Guide to Good Practice in the Care of Individuals with Long-term Mental Health Disorders. No. 4.

[15] Kingdon, D. Making Care Programming Work. *Advances in Psych Treatment; Vol.1, 41–44, 1994.*

[16] Jones, K., Robinson, M. & Golightley, P. Long-term psychiatric patients in the community. *Brit J Psych* 1986; **149**: 537–540.

8 Schizophrenia: Issues for General Practice

THOMAS MEREDITH DAVIES, Deputy Vice Chairman, Royal College of General Practitioners 1989–90

Background

The Government's White Paper 'Caring for People'[1], which addressed many of the problems faced by the schizophrenic patient and his/her family had almost become the 'forgotten' white paper, by the time of the Conference overshadowed by consideration of its 'companion', *Working for Patients*[2], and imposition of the new GP contract[3]. However, as this book shows, it may well be that *Caring for People* will have the greatest long-term effect on the GP and the primary health care team.

Caring for People

The Royal College of General Practitioners' response to the White Paper, highlighted concerns about many areas. Included were questions about resources, general principles of community care, problems with working together with different agencies and worries about assessment for care in the community. The College however welcomed the opportunity for professionals and voluntary groups to discuss each other's roles; to share opinions and ideas; and to thus try to reach a better mutual understanding about working together which would benefit patient or client. The College's clinical folder, 'Care for Schizophrenic patients and their families'[4] has been well received and will, I hope, find a place in most GPs' libraries.

For too long, the treatment of schizophrenia was seen as the exclusive province of the psychiatrists and a matter for hospitals. Studies of patients with schizophrenia in the community showed that up to one quarter were managed only by the primary care team[5]. The closure of Mental Hospitals, better use of drugs, and better training of community staff have all encouraged the development of care in the community. These changes should be supported, but unfortunately still too many patients discharged to community care risk ending up homeless, or in hostels in the bigger cities and lost to follow up. Richard Stone[6] has calculated in his practice area that there could be some 250 single people suffering from a mental illness in bed-and-breakfast accommodation.

One of the problems with the public's perception of schizophrenia is the bad press and media coverage it attracts. Sensationalism helps no one. There is undoubtedly still a major stigma attached to the diagnosis of schizophrenia

79

and major misunderstanding of the treatments available (see chapter 4) and the long term prognosis. One per cent of the population will be diagnosed as schizophrenic at some time in their lives. Most patients present at the prime of their lives, namely between 16 and 25 years of age. Anthony Clare suggested[7] that 80 per cent of women and 60 per cent of men recover from acute episodes, sufficiently well enough to return to normal functions in the community. The GP and primary health care team has a crucial role to play: both to help individuals and their carers, and to put to rest the various myths which have abounded for years.

GPs: The first point of contact

A GP with an average list size (eg 2300) may expect to diagnose one new schizophrenic a year, and be responsible for three chronic cases. Of all health and social care workers, he or she is the most likely to have known the family over the longest time up to 30–35 years. The GP thus has a key role to play, with other members of the primary health care team, in the diagnosis and management of this disabling illness. The GP will, in most cases of schizophrenia, be the point of first contact for the patient and his/her relatives. Diagnosis is obviously crucial, but treatment may be started without a firm diagnosis. Indeed delay can make things worse. A consultant psychiatrist should be involved—often with a domiciliary visit—and hospital admission might be necessary.

Relatives who are often also the GP's patients, should be party to all decisions regarding patient care. The GP will often need to spend a lot of time explaining the illness, and dealing with what in many ways is similar to a bereavement reaction (see Chapter Two). Relatives need to address and resolve their denial, anger and guilt. They will want answers to unanswerable questions, "Why did this happen?", and "Why to us"? They may be done a disservice by speculation over the years that environmental factors have been a significant cause of the illness.

The GP has undoubtedly an increasingly important role in helping prevent the breakdown of interpersonal and inter-family relationships. Successful rehabilitation of the patient, including those with schizophrenia, is more likely with family support. Whilst patients are in hospital, their GP should be kept abreast of progress.

Hospital Care

Admission

Hospital admission may occur on an voluntary or involuntary basis. The change in the Mental Health Act in 1983, created some problems for GPs, particularly in the interpretation of Sections 2 and 3: that a person may be admitted to hospital in the interests of his or her own health as well as for his or her own safety or for the protection of other persons. This has often been interpreted as confined to the physical safety, but such an unnecessarily restricted view can cause great distress, and deny the patient essential treatment.

Discharge

Hospital discharge is the key area. Over 50 per cent of people who have been treated for schizophrenia in hospital will be discharged to the care of a relative[8]. There must be the closest collaboration with *all* concerned *prior* to discharge. Indeed, at the time the patient is admitted to hospital, the GP should have some plan for the long term aim in treatment and the preferred place of discharge. Discharge should not be premature and be fully discussed with the primary care team. Complete understanding is required about:–

Who continues to have the overall clinical responsibility

Who is providing/administering the treatment

Who is following up the patient

What agencies are involved in the care

Clinical responsibility after discharge from hospital

As regards the question, "Who continues to have the overall clinical responsibility?" the Royal College of General Practitioners firmly believes that the care of any person in the community is the responsibility of the *primary care physician* (GP) working in closest collaboration with the secondary care services (ie where hospital specialists may be involved). Kendrick[9] however reported that most GPs preferred the clinical responsibility to remain with the psychiatrist. For individual patients, plans must be explicit and known to everyone involved in their care. If the patient is to be discharged out of the referring GP's area or if the patient previously had no GP, arrangements should be made with a new GP, before discharge.

The community psychiatric nurse (CPN) is also a key person, whom the College would like to see far more closely integrated into the primary health care team. The CPN provides the link between the hospital and GP. Counselling skills may be all important, and in time, CPNs may even be altering drug dosages as appropriate.

General practice can give excellent care, but several authors have shown that for this group care can be improved. Nazareth[10] highlighted a deficiency in recording physical and mental health. There is a need for good and regular liaison with the local psychiatric services[11]. Kendrick[12] advocates the use of structured management plans, looking at issues such as continuity of care, social and physical assessments and modification of risk factors and specialist drug review. Training for all involved, doctors, team members and carers and patients is advised by Falloon.[13]

Shared Records

As patients continue to be increasingly looked after at home, by ever knowledgeable team, the need to share information will continue to be of the highest importance. Shared records, ideally to be used by medical, nursing, social workers, voluntary workers and carers will be an important thing to consider. Popular with patients, they were less popular with mental health professionals[14]. Taking the patient/client's and carer's views into account however will encourage a frank and honest dialogue for future care.

Supervision Registers

In response to several tragedies highlighted in the media the government in 1994 announced plans to set up supervision registers.[15] The aim of such a register was to keep contact with patients known 'to be at significant risk of committing serious violence or suicide or of serious self-neglect as a result of severe and enduring mental illness'. Professional concerns remain as to the medico-legal consequences of such a register and the time consuming and expensive independent inquiries that may be necessary for people involved with 'serious incidents of violence'.[16]

Conclusion

This brief introduction has hardly mentioned Social Services, or social workers. Implementation of *Caring for People* has given the latter overall responsibility for the administration and co-ordination of client's social and health care needs. This is not to forget the valuable counselling skills possessed by individual social workers. The new 'case managers' will also need tremendous support both financially and emotionally. The inevitable question is—will there be enough resources?

For a few patients, long term hospital care will remain the only realistic solution. The Royal College of General Practitioners believes that all such people, in hospitals or long term care for more than six months, should have access to the provision of primary care provided by a GP and primary health care team. These people still have long-term health care needs which, over the years, might easily have been or be forgotten.

References

[1] United Kingdom Secretaries of State for Health, Social Security, Wales and Scotland. *Caring for People: Community care in the next decade and beyond*. (CM 849). London: HMSO 1989.
[2] United Kingdom Secretaries of State for Hedalth, Wales Northern Ireland and Scotland. *Working for patients: The Health service: caring for 1990s*. (CM 555) London: HMSO 1989.
[3] Department of Health, Welsh Office and Scottish Office. *General Practice in the National Health Service: the 1990 contract*. London: HMSO 1989.
[4] Ryall, R., Kiupers, L., Steel, R., et al. Eds *Care for schizophrenic patients and their families*. (Information folder). London: RCGP 1990.
[5] Campbell G. P., Taylor J., Pantelis C., Harvey C. Studies of schizophrenia in a large mental hospital proposed for closure and in two halves of an inner London borough served by the hospital. In Weller M. (ed) International perspectives in schizophrenia: biological, social and epidemiological findings. London. John Libbey 1990.

6   Stone R. Chapter 7. General Practitioners, schizophrenia and homelessness. RCGP. *Care for schizophrenic patients and their families*. (Information folder). London: RCGP 1990.

7   Clare, A. Psychiatry in Dissent. 2nd Edition, London: Tavistock, 1980.

8   Ryall, R. Chapter 2: 'A overview of Schizophrenia' *Care for schizophrenic patients and their families*. (Information folder). London: RCGP 1990.

9   Kendrick T, Sibbald B, Burns T, Freeling P. Role of general practitioners in care of long term mentally ill patients. *British Medical Journal* 1991; **302**: 508–510.

10 Nazareth I. D., King M. Controlled evaluation of management of schizophrenia in one general practice: a pilot study. Family Practice 1992. 9(2): 171–2.

11 Boddington, J. Role of general practitioners in the care of the long term mentally ill. *British Journal of Psychiatry*, 1992 **160**: 568–9.

12 Kendrick T. Care of patients with schizophrenia. 1993 *British Journal of General Practice*. **43**: 259–260.

13 Falloon I. R., Shanahan W., Laporta M., Krekorian H. A., Integrated family, general practice and mental health care in the management of schizophrenia. 1990. *Journal of the Royal Society of Medicine* **83 (4)**225–8.

14 Essex B., Doig R., Renshaw J. Pilot study of records of shared care for people with a mental illness. *British Medical Journal* 1990; **300**: 1442–1446.

15 NHS Management Executive *Introduction of supervision registers for mentally ill patients from 1 April 1994*. Leeds. NHSME 1991 (HSG(94)5).

16 Harrison G., Barlett B., Supervision registers for mentally ill people. *British Medical Journal* 1994; **309**: 551–2.

9 The Role of the Family Health Services Authority in Assessing Need and Distributing Resources

JOHN JAMES, *formerly* General Manager, Kensington and Chelsea and Westminster Family Health Service Authority

SUMMARY

Family Health Services Authorities (FHSAs) have a role in helping general practitioners and other members of the primary care team to extend preventive and health promotion activities in the area of mental health, particularly in the inner cities where mental health problems are more prevalent. Methods of implementing change may involve training initiatives for primary care team members, education of team members in the understanding and treatment of people with mental health problems, and the provision of adequate back-up and support work from other statutory and voluntary agencies, including additional support staff for practices directly funded by the FHSA. This paper briefly discusses how the Kensington and Chelsea and Westminster Family Health Services Authority is working with general practitioners and primary health care workers in the area to ensure that resources are targeted where health needs are greatest.

Background

The opportunity to address the conference on mental health and primary care came at a time when the National Health Service and in particular Family Practitioner Committees (FPCs)—now called Family Health Services Authorities (FHSAs) were undergoing major changes. I suspect that a few years ago it would have been unlikely for an FPC administrator to address such a conference on the topics of assessing need and distributing resources.

At the time this presentation was made, responsibility for administering general practice (and other primary care services) had just shifted from Family Practitioner Committees (FPCs) to Family Health Services Authorities (FHSAs). The latter were charged with a broader role than FPCs had been in planning and commissioning quality primary care services for their local populations. Responsibility for commisssioning acute and community services rested with District Health Authorities (DHAs). Since then, yet more changes have occurred. FHSAa have combined with DHAs to form new, integrated Authorities. Their ability to allocate additional resources to those practices with higher numbers of patients with severe mental illness has, therefore, been further enhanced.

The Family Practitioner Health Service Authority Area

The area of Kensington and Chelsea and Westminster has significant pockets of wealth, but it also has pockets of deprivation and problems unique to the inner city. In particular, there are increasing levels of homelessness and mental health problems in the community. Against this background, FPCs (and the new FHSAs) have to establish primary health care services in their localities, of a range and quality which enable access and equality and not discriminate against the less able or articulate members of the community. This never has been an easy task and will provide a challenge for everyone involved in commissioning health services and providing primary health care for the foreseeable future. Commissioning community health services provides a similar challenge for purchasers.

Needs assessment and resource allocation

One of the ways of measuring how well FHSAs do in the short term will be how well we apply our limited resources to support general practice in dealing with problems of mental health and homelessness in the community. The end aim is to meet the health needs and to seek improvement in health status; thus the role of the FHSAs on assessing needs and distributing resources is a critical new area of activity.

In the past, although FPCs did not **have** to assess health needs and allocate cash-limited resources in this way, some did. Their good work and innovation should be applauded.

Roles for the Family Health Services Authority

The new FHSA has three main roles:

(i) As an authority charged with the administration of family health services.

(ii) As an authority charged with the management, planning and policy role for primary health care services in collaboration with other statutory and voluntary organisation; and

(iii) As an employing authority, like any other employing authority: eg, district health authority or local authority.

Administration (i) formed essentially the largest proportion of the FPCs' work prior to April 1985. The organisation's work was largely prescribed in detail (eg, complaints, payments).

FPCs had—indeed, FHSAs still have—some degree of discretion. Management discretion towards developing new and appropriate services will largely rest on how imaginative FHSAs are prepared to be, and how flexible they are prepared to be with GPs about particular local service issues.

The past role of the FPC in service planning and development is a key area for future work by FHSAs. There will be much more emphasis on assessing need and allocating resources; generally bringing about the need for much more robust management and development of local services. If these areas are not handled effectively and efficiently, we will not make any real impact on service improvements—particularly in inner-city areas.

National Health Service reforms

One of the aims of the NHS reforms is to provide a better deal for the patient. Synonymous with a better deal will be the FHSAs' responsibility to target resources where health need is greatest. In an inner city area—with high population mobility, different facets of homelessness, and primary mental health problems—it is for FHSAs, and district health authority purchasers and providers to ensure that the NHS reforms are translated into better services for these groups.

There is a quite clear emphasis on health promotion and illness prevention within the broad thrust of the documents. However, there is a real danger, if care is not taken, that more time will be spent on health promotion activity for the 'worried well'—not for people in greatest need in the community.

Information suggests that ethnic minority groups are over-represented in the mentally-ill sector. This is a worrying trend and suggests the need for more appropriate community-based health initiatives.

Joint working

FPCs/FHSAs must work together with general practices towards positive action. The Kensington & Chelsea & Westminster FHSA has embarked on a collaborative process with local GPs and district health authority (DHA) departments of public health, collecting and disseminating data from GP annual health reports. This, we believe, will go some way towards developing joint health profiles of the local population. We would then want to agree, with the GPs and DHAs, health priorities and targets. We will therefore target resources to certain practices as appropriate. Experience has shown however, that practices willing to produce a full range of services are sometimes overwhelmed because nearby practices do not want to accept their share of responsibility.

Two examples of successful liaison in our area are:

(i) A GP in the Kensington and Chelsea and Westminster area is involved in a project we implemented locally in collaboration with the voluntary sector (Family Welfare Association). A social support post is jointly funded by the FHSA and FWA to deal with particular social issues within a practice. A large component of this work involves supporting patients with mental health problems.

(ii) A group practice in Bayswater, working with the management of the project from the FPC, collectively decided to share the responsibility for providing primary health care to homeless families in temporary accommodation in the Bayswater area[1,2]. The scheme works with a rota of about 12 GPs who each gives sessional time and are supported by a practice nurse.

Another way of providing 'hands-on' support for practices is by way of well-trained support staff, either directly funded by FPCs, or via the district health authorities and the voluntary sector.

Conclusion

The NHS reforms really do have to be used and applied imaginatively by FHSAs to ensure that the changes which have been put forward as part of the reforms can make real improvements to local services and the health status of the population. FHSAs must also encourage general practices to share the workload and support practice, both financially and otherwise, to bring about positive change.

References

[1] Dennis, H. *It's so good to know it's there: a preliminary review of the Bayswater Families Doctors Practice.* London: Kensington, Chelsea & Westminster Family Health Services Authority, 1990.

[2] Simon Hope. Caring for the homeless. *RCGP Connection* 1991; **April:** 2–3.

Address for contact

John James, Divisional General Manager, Kings Healthcare NHS Trust, Denmark Hill, London SE5 9RS.

10 Schizophrenia and the Primary Care Team: A Regional Perspective

PETER CLARKE, Chief Executive, Mental Health Services of Salford
HILARY HODGE, Director of Priority Services, North West Region

SUMMARY

Current mental health policy is moving from a reliance on large mental hospitals towards district psychiatric services which provide an integrated range of primary and specialist care. In this context health regions have a key role in stimulating and monitoring the purchasing decisions of health purchasers prompting a collaborative approach between the health purchasers, local authorities and other agencies. They also have a role in ensuring that proper attention is given to the development of relevant skills. Regions may be at a distant, strategic level within the organisational structure, but it is essential that the development of policy, the way it is monitored and the concern for skill development reflect the reality of schizophrenia as experienced by individuals and their families.

Background

I shall outline the nature of the Region's role in monitoring and skills development, against a background of the policy objectives.

Mental Health Policy

The large Victorian mental hospitals are clearly an affront. There is no conceivable justification for allowing them to continue unchanged, as parts of our mental health service. They must go, not as a means of saving money or from some kind of new whim, but in recognition that people who experience mental illness deserve better than can be offered by the deprivation of those hospitals.

There does seem to be a real danger that the policy commitment to service change may be highjacked by those who are seeking to free patients not from hospitals but from psychiatry. There is irony in this because it denies the pain and disorder of those who experience serious mental illness rather in the same way that some would argue that hospital deny individual rights. It is a dangerously powerful force, particularly when it is exploited by managers whose concerns are actually to make savings rather than to achieve service change. So, I am committed to the closure of large hospitals and I approach policy from that perspective, but I am concerned that we achieve it in a way which acknowledges the need for a new service and not merely the destruction of an old service. Policy now recognises this and there is a clear expectation that resources from hospital closures must be ring fenced to provide for the new community based care. The national policy was for districts to have a local psychiatric service based on psychiatric units located in District General Hospital Units. It is easy to see the large hospitals as all things evil and the modern DGH unit as all things desirable. However, DGH units can provide services which are as inappropriate for the individuals who use them as the large hospitals. Neither necessarily do what is required. Neither reach into the nature of the mental illness and provide an appropriate means to enable users achieve relevant outcomes.

Mental illness may be seen to have two inextricably linked components.

(i) an internal disorder of thoughts, perceptions and feelings and

(ii) an external disruption of social roles and relationships.

It is not possible to separate these. It is not in fact possible to separate health and social factors, they are integral parts of the one experience. The services must address both dimensions and recognise the interplay between each: to do this effectively, the service environment and the service culture need themselves to be therapeutic. They inevitably have a significant impact upon the outcome of the treatment.

The policy which Regions must ensure is implemented therefore has to ensure that new service systems are developed which:

(i) reflect the reality of the complex needs of the individual;

(ii) build on the best leading edge of skills and understanding of mental illness;

(iii) operate in a way which acknowledges the full complex of a dynamic treatment process.

Policy cannot be simply about closing large hospitals; it must create a new pattern of service.

Monitoring

We are all struggling to understand the details of the forms of patterns of service which can achieve this. Examples of good practice are infrequent although increasing but are still partial: most of us are still at the crawling stage. We have much to learn before we can run. However, it is clear that development of new patterns of service will cross boundaries between primary and specialist care. Primary care services have a crucial role to play in a full response to the needs of people with schizophrenia. The tragedy to date is that, too often, they have abdicated their responsibilities in favour of the specialist services without recognising that it is inappropriate so to do. A range of services is required in which primary and secondary care both play a full part.

The development of a comprehensive and complex range of services will require resources, whether these be new in nature or a new use of old resources. Current deficiencies in primary care cannot be 'made good' without new resources.

Region must ensure the protection of the existing level of resources allocated for mental health services: "Ring Fencing", for example ensures that the current spend committed to mental health services is an *irreducible minimum* not a ceiling.

Historically, the North Western Region attempted to ring fence resources. As the changes in methods of allocation occur then all Regions will need to develop a much more sophisticated approach to tracking resources which should be devoted to mental health through their new performance management role.

Regions will need to develop more subtle means of achieving policy objectives: performance management and monitoring will be a key tool, and they will need to look very carefully at the purchasing and other decisions of health purchasers, will assess the health (including mental health) needs of their population and will then make judgements about the appropriate service response to those needs. It is relatively easy to identify the level of need, but very much more difficult to make the rationing judgements. These determine which services an authority can afford to deliver and which it cannot (or chooses not to).

In this particular field, whilst lessons are learned about new forms of service, it can also be difficult to identify the nature of the service response needed. Regions will have to monitor purchasing decisions, holding authorities to account for the reasons why they might have chosen, for example, not to develop services for people with schizophrenia. They will also need to ensure that purchasing decisions result in the development of services which benefit the mentally ill and their families.

Regions have another monitoring role: The *Community Care Plans*[1] which are developed by local authorities in conjunction with health purchasers. This is one of the means by which the purchasing intentions of health purchasers and the plans of local authorities are explicitly integrated in order to reduce the risk of a gap developing between *health* and *social* care—and people with chronic mental illness would tend to be the casualty of any such gaps. Regions will need to continue monitoring the strategies as they are established and updated by purchasing authorities at a local level, in order to ensure that there is a coherence across the agencies. They will be seeking evidence that there is a consistent strategy of development to deliver the relevant resources and that this is delivered through effective use of the *Individual Care Programme Approach*[2]. Again, the impact upon the lives of users and their carers will be the key concern.

Regions in connection with purchasers also have a significant, albeit more limited, monitoring role at a provider level. The Individual Care Programme approach is an important component of mental health care, especially when linked to the *Care Management*[3] Systems run by LAs. RHAs need to ensure that continued development work takes place in care management and the more recently introduced Supervision Register. If the Care Programme Approach is to really help people cope with the personal distress and disorder imposed by mental illness, regions will need to identify ways of asking questions which show that health purchasers are applying the approach effectively ie, satisfying the needs of clients. Individual care programmes cannot be concerned only with specialist and secondary levels of care: they must include as an integral ingredient, the contributions made by relevant primary care workers.

One specific aspect of RHAs need to monitor when they look at the strategies and purchasing decisions (as well as when they look at the development of care programmes), is the way in which the component parts fit together. Of key importance are mechanisms which enable staff to communicate effectively: and so bring reality to the notions of team work and multidisciplinary and interagency collaboration.

Regions cannot be involved with the operational detail of service provision, but their monitoring must be broad and deep enough to ensure they know what is actually being developed for people with schizophrenia and their families. They will need to ensure they have up-to-date and relevant knowledge about "best practice" and of the real constraints within which services operate.

The development and subsequent expansion of GP Fundholding has accompanied a shift in the centre of gravity of the NHS as it becomes Primary Care Led. In the context of mental health services there is currently little evidence of how the purchasing power of GPs will impact upon what is available to people with schizophrenia and serious mental illnesses. There is, however, some evidence of a tension between the national policy priorities reflected in the Supervision Register and supervised discharge legislation, on the one hand and the pressures felt by GPs from people whose needs are for counselling and short term support. Traditionally, the secondary services have absorbed, and to some extent hidden, those with substantial and sustained needs. Health Purchasers will need to develop a market management capacity whilst the Region will monitor the emerging situation.

Skill development

Regions may help shape services by focusing on the policy and by monitoring purchasing strategies. They can have further impact by helping develop a knowledge base in primary care—one which would include both the particular skills needed by primary care staff to intervene appropriately in the lives of people with schizophrenia, and also, the understanding of schizophrenia which primary care workers need in order to discuss it clearly with others. GPs and other primary care staff have an important role in a new pattern of services where increasing numbers of mentally ill people are living in the community with a support system to sustain them. GPs are key components of that support system and must have clinical skills appropriate for their role.

Skills in communication and understanding are of perhaps equal importance. Many people close to the patient are adversely affected by the onset of schizophrenia: many have a sense of ignorance, frustration and fear. They have a right to expect help with coming to terms with the illness confronting them. If they can be helped to do this, they will be better able to provide appropriate levels of support, and less likely to compound existing problems. Regions have a role in ensuring that health purchasers support GPs and other workers in primary care to develop the specialist knowledge and skills required for this education/communication task—as well as direct interaction.

Conclusion

The process of setting up a policy framework for developing, monitoring and influencing skills development must be part of the whole dynamic for improvement in the essence of mental health care. Regions should not be preoccupied solely with the external appurtenances of services, such as the numbers of beds or levels of resources. Those are important, but Regions should actually be touching on how services are working and how they are experienced by the users and carers. This is where the essence of mental health care lies.

From my perspective, I see no place for any dramatic declaration by Regions of a new pattern of service. But neither is there any place for an absence of vision or a denial of the 'awfulness' of much of the current service. Life may never come right for people who experience schizophrenia, but primary care services have a key role in helping them to cope, adjust, and manage their problems. Regions must ensure that the environment within which the primary and specialist services work is consistent with these aspirations. This requires their performance management monitoring processes to be informed by both reality and a vision of what the services must be if they are effectively and efficiently to meet needs.

When this paper was first contributed the author was Director of Community Services, North Western Region. It has been updated in collaboration with Dr Hilary Hodge, Director, Priority Services, North West Region.

References

1. Department of Health. *Caring for People: community care in the next decade and beyond*. London: HMSO, 1989 (Cm 849).
2. Department of Health. *The Care Programme Approach for People with a mental illness referred to the specialist psychiatric services*. Heywood (Lancashire): Department of Health 1990 (Health Circular: HC(90)23/LASSL(90)11).
3. Department of Health. *Caring for People: community care in the next decade and beyond*. London: HMSO, 1989. (Cm 849).

Address for contact

Peter Clark, Chief Executive, Mental Health Services of Salford, Bury New Road, Prestwich, Manchester M25 3BL.

11 The Shift to Community Mental Health Care: The Impact on General Practitioners

TONY KENDRICK, Senior Lecturer in General Practice and Primary Care, St George's Hospital Medical School

SUMMARY

A survey of general practitioners (GPs) in SW Thames region found that only 30% had noticed an effect of the discharge of adult long-term mentally ill (LTMI) patients on their practices: the majority estimated that they each had 10 or fewer such patients on their lists. Having higher estimated numbers was significantly associated with practising in Greater London; practising near a large mental hospital; and having contact with a psychiatrist visiting the practice. Most GPs were willing to share the care of LTMI patients with the consultant psychiatrist, by taking responsibility for physical problems, with the community psychiatric nurse as key worker. Very few practices had any specific policies for the care of the LTMI.

A more detailed study has since been carried out in 16 group practices in SW Thames. A total of 440 LTMI patients were identified, a prevalence of 3 per 1000. Only two thirds were in current contact with psychiatric teams, whilst over 90% were seen frequently by their GPs, mainly for physical problems and sickness certificates. Teaching the general practitioners a structured assessment to use with their LTMI patients was associated with a subsequent increase in psychotropic drug changes and referrals to specialist teams.

Background

The move to community care

Since its peak in the mid–1950s, the psychiatric inpatient population has been steadily falling, with the closure of some hospitals and reduction of beds by three quarters in many others (see Chapter Three). Patients who in the past might have become long-stay residents are now much more likely to be discharged.

Despite advances in treatment, however, many mentally ill people still require support on a long-term basis. For example, 40–50 per cent of patients with schizophrenia have residual symptoms and seriously impaired social functioning requiring long-term treatment.[1,2] (see Chapter 1).

Since 1975, Government policy has been to run down and close the old large mental hospitals, replacing them with a local network of health and social services in each district, including general hospital psychiatric departments, day hospitals, community psychiatric services, and local authority residential, day care and social work support services.[3]

Over 100,000 psychiatric beds in England have been closed.[4] However, the provision of community facilities such as day hospitals and day centres has not been accomplished at the same rate.[5] There is therefore an increasing number of long-term mentally ill (LTMI) patients living outside hospital, and only a minority of them are likely to be attending day facilities.

Responsibility for the long-term mentally ill

Most patients leaving hospital after their first admission for a serious psychiatric illness like schizophrenia are young adults who often return to their families, and to the care of their family doctor. A study by Parkes *et al* in South London in the early 1960s suggested that such patients relied heavily on their general practitioner (GP) for day-to-day medical care.[6] Whilst over 70 per cent of the patients saw their GPs regularly, only 60 per cent were followed in psychiatric outpatients, and half of those were seen less than five times in the year after discharge. Most GP consultations were brief contacts, for repeat prescriptions and sickness certificates. However, when the patient's mental state deteriorated, it was usually the GP who was involved initially, rather than the psychiatrist.

Concurrent with the move to community care, there has been an increase in the number of psychiatrists who treat patients in general practice settings,[7] including patients with both psychotic and chronic disorders.[8,9] In some areas, case registers of long-term patients have been maintained by the psychiatric services, and some community mental health teams make strenuous efforts to keep in contact with the long-term mentally ill.[10] However it is apparent, at least in South London, that the general practitioner is still very much involved in the care of such patients after hospital discharge, even more frequently than the psychiatrist. In 1991 Melzer *et al* found that, 12 months after discharge, whilst 52% of patients were attending psychiatric outpatients, 57% had been in recent contact with their GPs.[11]

The Royal College of Psychiatrists recommended that consultants should be responsible for keeping up-to-date registers of long-term mentally ill patients and should delegate their responsibility for community care only to a named key worker.[12] Discharge to GP care should happen only when aftercare is no longer necessary. This was made official Government policy in the Care Programme Approach,[13] specifying that before hospital discharge, all vulnerable patients must have a named key worker and a written care plan, which must be communicated to all the professionals likely to be involved in a person's care, including their GP.

Shared care

Even if patients continue under psychiatric supervision, they are entitled to GP care. The Royal College of General Practitioners stressed that GPs are legally responsible under their terms of service for patients registered with them[14]. A working party of the two Royal Colleges urged that GPs and psychiatrists should work more closely together, and made a number of recommendations for shared care.[15] They suggested that psychiatrists should spend some of their time working on GPs' premises, help GPs to set up registers of their vulnerable long-term mentally ill patients, agree guidelines for treatment and referral, and take part in mutual training and joint audit.

Fig 11.1: *SW Thames Region inpatient data for mental illness*

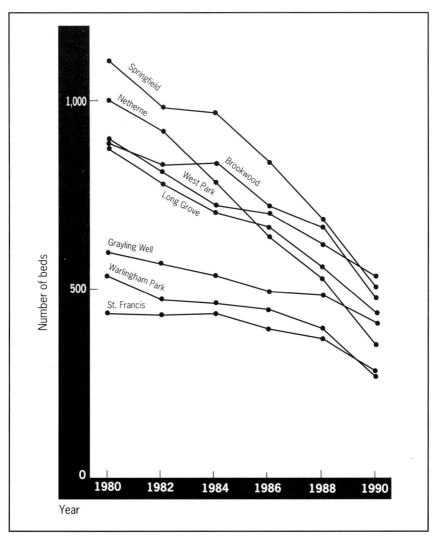

However Ben Essex, in a study of the feasibility of patient-held shared care record cards, suggested that many doctors, specialists and GPs alike, might not be keen on shared care.[16] Elizabeth Horder reported that psychiatrists responsible for the placement of long-stay residents sometimes found they had to persuade one or two of the more interested local GPs to take on the primary care needs of all the residents of a group home or hostel, rather than sharing them out.[17]

Whether they like it or not, GPs cannot ignore long-term mentally ill patients who decline to attend the psychiatric day hospitals and fail to turn up to outpatients. Those who do attend are the responsibility of the GP at night and weekends. Patients move house and are lost to hospital follow-up. For example, in a community survey in south Camden, only 60 per cent of patients suffering from chronic schizophrenia were found to be in current contact with psychiatric services.[18]

The GP's contact with a large proportion of the population means he or she is in a good position to identify people with mental illness who are unknown to the psychiatric or social services, and therefore in danger of 'slipping through the net'.

A model for community care

The Department of Health and Social Security funded a Medical Research Council study to evaluate a model programme of community care in Worcester. This involved the closure of an old asylum, Powick, and the provision of two general hospital psychiatric units, four day hospitals, four psychiatric day centres and two psychiatric hostels in its place.[19] The study reported that most local GPs thought the services were an improvement and were satisfied with the care provided for their patients. Only 20 per cent thought that their workload had increased as a result of the changes.

However, the development in Worcester was a well-funded demonstration project. Concern has been expressed that community care is not working very well in many other areas. Considerable difficulties reported include a lack of suitably-trained social workers prepared to work with the mentally ill, and competing demands on Social Services (eg. children on the at-risk register). A shortage of appropriate housing has left discharged patients lacking suitable accommodation. In 1989, Marshall recorded that many disabled former residents of long-stay wards, with residual symptoms, were living in hostels in Oxford, unsupported by psychiatrically-trained staff;[20] a third of destitute men in the Crisis at Christmas Inner London Survey (1985–88) were found to be suffering from hallucinations and delusions;[21] and in 1984, a disproportionately high percentage of men with schizophrenia was found among those on remand in Brixton prison.[22]

Most recently, great public concern has arisen over the potential for self-harm or violence, highlighted by the actions of Ben Silcock and Christopher Clunis, and led to calls for greater supervision of people with serious mental health problems after discharge from hospital. The report of enquiry into the treatment of Christopher Clunis[23] suggested a national register should be set up of people who have been repeatedly compulsorily admitted or who are at serious risk of violence, repeated offending, or homelessness. The Health Secretary's 10–point plan for the supervision of discharged patients, whilst eschewing the idea of a national register, did propose plans for district-based supervision registers, which are being implemented at the time of writing.[24]

A significant minority of LTMI patients are not registered with GPs.[25] In cases where community care is not working, GPs might not have increasing numbers of LTMI patients on their lists, simply because the patients are homeless and have not registered with a practice.

How many disabled patients per GP?

Inpatient numbers in my health region, South West Thames (now South Thames West), fell by something like 8,000 between 1960 and 1980. The initial drop was due both to the deaths of older, long-stay residents and to the discharge of the rather less-disabled, more independent patients. However, as bed reductions continued, more and more symptomatic and disabled patients had to be considered for discharge. Figure 11.1 shows the continued contraction of the inpatient population of the South West (SW) Thames Region: another 3,000 or so beds went between 1980 and 1990. Approximately 500 psychiatric beds were provided in district general hospital units, but they remained constant throughout the 1950s and were not used for the long-term mentally ill.

To put these figures into perspective: approximately 1500 GPs practise in the SW Thames Region, so on average, each GP would be likely to have had an increase of only a handful of LTMI patients on his or list. In practice, of course the distribution of such patients might not be uniform.

GPs with more than their share of the long-term mentally ill

I was struck by the fact that, in my former practice in Weybridge, in the stock-broker belt', I had not noticed an effect of the discharge of patients who in the past were, or might have been, kept in long-stay wards. There were no hostels or group homes where I practised, and I thought I could count the number of LTMI patients on my own list on the fingers of one hand.

Speaking to GPs who practised in London, I heard a different story. One doctor, whose surgery is around the corner from a large mental hospital, told me that, in 1980, he agreed to take on to his list the residents of a new group home — a converted house. These patients had been living in the hospital for varying periods; some for over 40 years. At first, a social worker visited the house regularly and the patients attended psychiatric outpatients. After a while, however, the social worker stopped visiting and a change of consultant at the hospital seemed to result in many of the outpatient attendances stopping also. The GP felt that the house was kept going largely by the work of one of the residents, an ex-long-stay patient who was rather better at coping than the others.

The GP continued to prescribe long-term medication, which in many cases was possibly overdue for review, but he did not feel able to make decisions himself about whether or not to change the drug treatments. He tended to see the residents of the group home only when there was a crisis, which meant he often had to ask for repeated readmissions. He estimated that another 10 or so patients in local bedsits and residential homes were chronically psychiatrically ill, and overall it seemed that he had 15 or 20 such people on his list (ie. three or four times as many as I did).

I felt that relying on my recollection of LTMI patients on my list would tend to underestimate their number, so I looked for more. I systematically listed all the patients on repeat prescriptions for major tranquillisers, lithium, anticholinergics, and long-term antidepressants; plus those who were listed on the practice computer as suffering from schizophrenia or manic-depressive illness. This survey revealed 35 patients between five partners: my own list included only seven; two more than I could recall initially.

A survey of GPs in the SW Thames Region

As a result of this enquiry, we at St George's decided to survey GPs in our region, to determine how many had noticed an impact on their practices of the move to community care, and what role they saw for themselves in the management of long-term mentally ill patients in the community. We asked the following questions:

1. How many LTMI patients do GPs estimate they have on their lists?

2. Where are the GPs who have higher numbers of such patients? In the city? .... Next to a mental hospital?

3. Do GPs have policies or protocols in their practices which provide for anticipatory or preventive care of the LTMI?

4. Whose responsibility do GPs think such patients are: the psychiatrist's? .... the GP's? .... Social Services'?

Method

We designed a questionnaire to include these queries and sent it to every third general practitioner on the Family Health Services Authorities' lists for the South West Thames region. It was concerned only with the adult LTMI; we specifically excluded elderly, mentally impaired patients and mentally handicapped patients.

Two terms defined for the GPs were:

(i) Long-term mentally ill patients:

A group which includes patients with chronic schizophrenia or other psychosis, severe personality disorder, or severe neurosis, and who, by definition, require long term supervision.

(ii) Key worker

The person identified as the point of first contact for a patient, maintaining a central therapeutic relationship, assessing the person's needs and the needs of their carers, and acting to ensure the necessary help is received from the various statutory and voluntary bodies involved.

Results

At the time of the conference (July 1990) interim results of this survey were presented, based on the responses of the first 296 (56%) respondents. Of 507 GPs surveyed, 369 (73%) eventually replied. The final results were published in the British Medical Journal in March 1991[26], and are reproduced below, with the kind permission of the Journal.

Table 11.1: *Estimated numbers of LTMI* patients on GP's lists in SW Thames Region 1990*

Number of LTMI on each GP's list	GP respondents	
	Number	(%)
0–5	102	(27.6)
6–10	123	(33.3)
11–15	45	(12.2)
16+	56	(15.2)
Don't know	43	(11.7)

*LTMI: Long-term mentally ill patients

GPs' involvement with the LTMI

One hundred and ten respondents (30%) had noticed an effect of the discharge from hospital of long-term mentally ill patients on their practices, 79 specifically mentioning an increase in workload. The number of long-term mentally ill patients that general practitioners estimated they had on their lists is shown in Table 11.1.

Eighty GPs (22%) had experience of working in a hospital psychiatric post, and six (1.6%) were currently working part time in psychiatry. Only nine (2.4%) had specific practice policies for managing LTMI patients.

GPs' attitudes towards the care of LTMI patients

Most of the general practitioners preferred the patients to remain the prime clinical responsibility of the psychiatrist, although shared care was agreeable to the large majority. Over 90% were willing to be specifically responsible for detecting and managing the physical problems of the patients. The community psychiatric nurse was the person preferred as key worker, by 83%; only 16% agreed that the general practitioner should have this role. Most of the respondents thought that long-term mentally ill patients posed many problems for a practice. Half of the general practitioners, however, considered these patients to be better off out of hospital, and over half disagreed that they had a poor prognosis whatever was done for them.

Fig 11.2: *South West Thames Region*

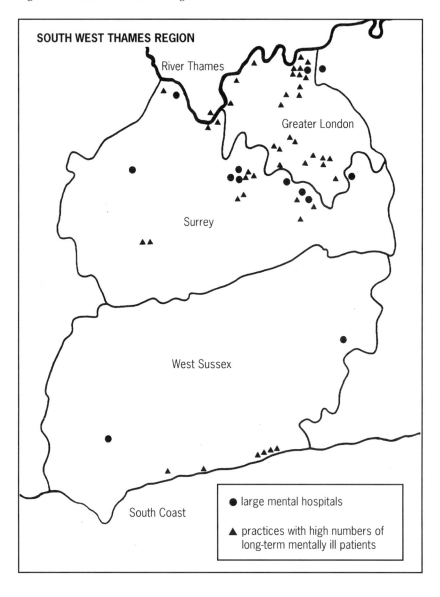

The higher the estimated number of long-term mentally ill patients the more likely was a general practitioner to be practising in Greater London; to be located within three miles of a large mental hospital (see Figure 11.2); have previous experience in a hospital psychiatry post; and have contact with a psychiatrist visiting the practice.

Conclusions

In most areas of the SW Thames Region, GPs have only a small number of LTMI patients on their lists. Only a minority report an increase in workload due to the move to community care.

It is not surprising that general practitioners with higher-than-average numbers of LTMI patients are more likely to:

(i) practise in London, and near large mental hospitals;

(ii) have worked in hospital psychiatry posts, and

(iii) have contact with a psychiatrist visiting their practices.

This supports the impression that, in practice, the consultant uses personal contact to persuade the more sympathetic local GPs to take onto their lists patients who, in the past would have remained in long-stay wards.

Most of the GPs surveyed said that they were ready to look after the physical problems, but preferred the pyschiatrist to keep overall responsibility, with the CPN acting as the key worker. Very few GPs had organised any protocols or policies for anticipatory care of the long-term mentally ill on their lists. We hypothesised that, if they could be helped to set up *programmes of systematic review*, they might avoid seeing such disadvantaged people only when there is a crisis, and the GP care of the LTMI would be improved. In the four years since the postal survey, we have examined this hypothesis, in more detailed work on the GP care of the LTMI.

Provision of care to general practice patients with disabling long-term mental illnesses: a survey in 16 practices.[27]

We set out to investigate the care of the LTMI in more detail, by setting up case registers in 16 group general practices. A search of each practice's record systems (including repeat prescription systems, diagnostic indices, appointment and visit books) was combined with a survey of local psychiatric and social service teams, to seek patients of the practice who might not be identified from the general practice data. We defined as long-term mentally ill those with enduring disability due to impaired social behaviour associated with mental illness, rather than selecting patients with a specific psychiatric diagnosis such as schizophrenia.

Practice records of the LTMI patients were examined for psychiatric diagnoses, the number and content of general practitioner consultations recorded within the preceding 12 months, and for indications of contacts with psychiatrists, community psychiatric nurses, or social workers in correspondence received.

Table 11.2 *Recorded diagnoses of the long-term mentally ill and their contacts with professionals*

Diagnosis recorded in GP files	Number of patients	No. (%) seen by their GPs in the last 12 months	No. of GP consultations per year (mean)	Number (%) currently in contact with:				Number (%) ever in contact with psychiatrists
				psychiatrists	CPNs	Either psychiatrists or CPNs	social workers	
Schizophrenia/ Schizo-affective disorder	204	181 (89)	6.3	116 (57)	88 (43)	144 (70)	15 (7)	204 (100)
Manic-depressive psychosis	38	37 (97)	9.1	32 (84)	8 (21)	33 (87)	1 (3)	38 (100)
Psychotic depression	11	10 (91)	5.3	8 (73)	4 (36)	8 (73)	0	11 (100)
Total psychotic	253	228 (90)	6.6	155 (61)	100 (40)	185 (73)	16 (6)	253 (100)
Anxiety/depression	103	101 (98)	9.0	41 (40)	18 (17)	50 (48)	3 (3)	93 (91)
Agoraphobia	27	27 (100)	10.0	8 (30)	4 (15)	11 (41)	2 (7)	22 (81)
Personality disorder (no other diagnosis)	16	15 (93)	10.6	8 (50)	4 (25)	8 (50)	2 (12)	16 (100)
Alcohol abuse	15	15 (100)	18.3	9 (60)	5 (33)	9 (60)	1 (7)	14 (93)
Anorexia nervosa	7	7 (100)	9.6	4 (57)	1 (14)	4 (57)	0	7 (100)
Chronic atypical (psychogenic) pain	6	6 (100)	14.7	0	0	0	1 (17)	4 (67)
Obsessive-compulsive disorder	5	4 (80)	5.4	3 (60)	1 (20)	3 (60)	0	5 (100)
Drug abuse	4	4 (100)	5.5	1 (25)	0	1 (25)	1 (25)	4 (100)
Others	4	4 (100)	7.5	3 (75)	1 (75)	3 (75)	0	3 (75)
Total non-psychotic	187	183 (98)	10.0	77 (41)	33 (17)	89 (48)	10 (5)	168 (90)
TOTAL	440	411 (93)	8.1	232 (53)	133 (30)	276 (63)	26 (6)	421 (96)

Table 11.2 shows the main diagnoses recorded in the records, and the professional contacts of the LTMI patients identified. Over one third of the patients had no current contact with psychiatric services. Patients in contact with specialist care had been ill for a shorter time and were more likely to be suffering from psychotic illnesses. Over 90% of the patients had been seen by their general practitioners within 12 months, on average 8 times. Most consultations were for minor physical disorders, repeat prescriptions and sickness certificates. In a 12–month period, elements of the formal mental state examination were recorded in only one third of cases and adjustments of psychotropic medication in only one fifth. Similar findings were reported by Parkes *et al* back in 1963[6], and in a smaller study of patients with schizophrenia by Nazareth *et al*.[28]

We concluded that general practitioners could use their frequent contacts with their long-term mentally ill patients to play a greater role in monitoring the mental state and drug treatment of this group.

Increasing the involvement of GPs in the psychiatric care of the LTMI: a randomised controlled trial.[29]

The next phase of our study was a controlled evaluation of teaching GPs to carry out structured assessments of their LTMI, to determine whether such an approach was feasible and increased GP involvement in their patients' psychiatric care. In eight of the 16 practices previously studied, the GPs were trained to use a brief interview covering the mental state, social functioning and medication side effects, designed for use in ordinary surgery appointments every six months for two years. The impact on the process of care was measured by examining the patients' practice records. A random sample was interviewed in depth with the Present State Examination and Social Role Performance Schedule, to describe their characteristics for comparison with other studies of the long-term mentally ill.

Interviews with 101 of the LTMI patients found high levels of current symptoms and social disability, comparable to populations of patients in long-term psychiatric contact. After two years follow-up data were obtained on 85%. Of 171 intervention group patients, 73% received at least one structured GP assessment but only 15% received four assessments. The GPs reported that they found the assessments time-consuming in some cases, and did not feel that in themselves the assessments led to better care. However, changes in psychotropic medication, particularly neuroleptic drugs, and referrals for psychosocial problems, particularly to community psychiatric nurses, were significantly more frequent in the intervention group (Table 11.3).

Table 11.3 *Changes in psychotropic drug treatments and referrals after teaching GPs to carry out structured assessments of their LTMI* [29]

	Percentage of LTMI patients within practice whose treatment was changed (in 2 years)		Difference (Intervention minus Control)	Adjusted difference† (and 95% confidence intervals)
	Control Group n = 8 mean (and range)	Intervention Group n = 8 mean (and range)		
Changes of neuroleptic drugs	26.1 (16–47)	39.4 (17–52)	13.3	14.3 (4.3 to 24.3)**
Changes of antidepressant drugs	27.8 (17–44)	34.7 (18–53)	6.9	8.7 (–2.0 to 19.4)
Changes in other psychotropic drugs	23.2 (4–60)	37.8 (16–70)	14.6	16.0 (–3.4 to 35.5)
Any change in psychiatric drug treatment or dosage	51.4 (29–73)	66.9 (48–79)	15.5	16.6 (2.2 to 31.0)*
Referrals to Consultant Psychiatrists	15.1 (0–29)	21.7 (5–53)	6.6	11.6 (–4.9 to 28.1)
Referrals to Community Psychiatric Nurses	5.4 (0–21)	15.9 (0–32)	10.5	13.3 (2.0 to 24.6)*
Referrals to Social Services, Housing or Employment agencies	2.7 (0–13)	5.4 (0–17)	2.7	3.6 (–2.8 to 9.9)
Any type of referral for psychosocial problems	20.9 (0–42)	38.3 (13–68)	17.4	26.1 (7.9 to 44.3)*

† (adjusted for variation in activity prior to the intervention using multiple regression analysis).
* p < 0.05.
** p < 0.01.
LTMI Long-term mentally ill.

There were no significant differences found in admissions, self-harm, or use of the Mental Health Act, although the power of the study to detect differences in these less frequent events was very limited.

We concluded that GP structured assessments of their LTMI patients may lead to more drug treatment changes and increased referrals to mental health teams. However, even volunteer GPs were unable or unwilling to repeat such assessments on most of their LTMI patients at regular intervals.

Conclusions

Whether they like it or not, GPs are frequently involved in the care of the long-term mentally ill outside hospitals. The GP care of patients with disabling illnesses such as schizophrenia can be improved. GPs however are faced with many competing demands on their time. More training is required for most GPs, and increased resources are probably necessary before improvements in the GP of the long-term mentally ill can be generalised.

Acknowledgements

The author wishes to thank the following who have kindly given permission for the use of previously published material:

The Editors, British Journal of General Practice (reference 27 below) and British Medical Journal (reference 29 below).

References

1 Johnstone, E. C., Owens, D. G. C., Gold, A., Crow, T.J., MacMillon, J. F. Schizophrenic patients discharged from hospital – a follow-up study. *British Journal of Psychiatry*. 1984; **145**: 586–590.
2 Watt, D. C., Katz, K., Shepherd, M. The natural history of schizophrenia: a 5–year prospective follow-up of a representative sample of schizophrenics by means of a standardized clinical and social assessment. *Psychological Medicine* 1983; **13**: 663–670.
3 Department of Health and Social Security. *Better services for the mentally ill.* London: HMSO, 1975. (Cmnd.6233).
4 Thornicroft, G., Strathdee, G. How many psychiatric beds? *British Medical Journal* 1994; **309**: 970–971.
5 Audit Commission for Local Authorities in England and Wales. *Making a reality of community care.* London: HMSO, 1986.
6 Parkes, C. M., Brown, G. W., Monck, E. M. The General Practitioner and the schizophrenic patient. *British Medical Journal* 1962; **i**: 972–976.
7 Strathdee, G., Williams, P. A survey of psychiatrists in primary care: the silent growth of a new service. *Journal of the Royal College of General Practitioners.* 1984; **34**: 615–8.
8 Brown, R. M. A., Strathdee, G., Christie-Brown, J. R. W., Robinson, P. H. A comparison of referrals to primary care and hospital out-patient clinics. *British Journal of Psychiatry* 1988; **153**: 168–73.

9 Tyrer, P. Psychiatric clinics in general practice: an extension of community care. *British Journal of Psychiatry* 1984; **145**: 9–14.

10 McLean, E. K., Leibowitz, J. A. Towards a working definition of the long-term mentally ill. *Psychiatric Bulletin* 1989; **13**: 251–252.

11 Melzer, D., Hale, A. S., Malik , S. J., Hogman, G.A., Wood, S. Community care for patients with schizophrenia one year after hospital discharge. *British Medical Journal* 1991; **303**: 1023–1026.

12 Royal College of Psychiatrists. *Good practice in discharge and aftercare procedures for patients discharged from inpatient treatment.* London; Royal College of Psychiatrists 1989.

13 Department of Health . *The care programme approach for people with mental illness referred to the specialist psychiatric services.* Heywood; Department of Health 1990 (HC(90)23/LASSL(90)11).

14 Royal College of General Practitioners. *Comments on the working party report on good practice in discharge and aftercare procedures for patients discharged from inpatient treatment.* London: Royal College of General Practitioners 1990.

15 Royal College of General Practitioners. *Shared Care of Patients with Mental Health Problems.* (Occasional paper 60). London: Royal College of General Practitioners 1993.

16 Essex, B., Doig, R., Renshaw, J. Pilot study of records of shared care for people with mental illnesses. *British Medical Journal* 1990; **300**: 1442–1446.

17 Horder, E. *Medical care in three psychiatric hostels in Hampstead and Bloomsbury District Health Authority.* London: Hampstead and South Barnet GP Forum 1990.

18 Pantelis, C., Taylor, J., Campbell, P. The South Camden Schizophrenia Survey. An experience of community-based research. *Bulletin of the Royal College of Psychiatrists* 1988; **12**:98–101.

19 Bennet, C. The Worcester development project: general practitioner satisfaction with a new community psychiatric service. *Journal of the Royal College of General Practitioners* 1989; **39**:106–109.

20 Marshall, M. Collected and neglected: Are Oxford hostels for the homeless filling up with disabled psychiatric patients? *British Medical Journal* 1989; **299**:706–709.

21 Weller, M., Tobiansky, R. I., Hollander, D., Ibrahimi, S. Psychosis and destitution at Christmas 1985–1988. *Lancet* 1989; **2**:1509–1511.

22 Taylor, P. J., Gunn, J. Violence and psychosis. I–Risk of violence among psychotic men. *British Medical Journal* 1984; **288**:1945–1949.

23 Ritchie, J., Dick, D., Lingham, R. *The Report of the Inquiry into the Care and Treatment of Christopher Clunis.* London: HMSO, 1994.

24 Department of Health *Legislation planned to provide supervised discharge of psychiatric patients.* London: HMSO, 1993.

25 Shaw, J., Holloway, J. Who is your general practitioner? *British Medical Journal* 1991; **303**: 628.

26 Kendrick, T., Sibbald, B., Burns, T., Freeling, P. Role of general practitioners in care of long-term mentally ill patients. *British Medical Journal* 1991; **302**: 508–510.

27 Kendrick, T., Burns, T., Sibbald, B., Freeling, P. Provision of care to general practice patients with disabling long–term mental illness: a survey in 16 practices. *British Journal of General Practice.* 1994; **44**: 301–305.

[28] Nazareth, I., King, M., Haines, A., See Tai, S., Hall, G. Care of schizophrenia in general practice. *British Medical Journal* 1993; **307**: 910.

[29] Kendrick, T., Burns, T., Freeling, P. Randomised controlled trial of teaching GPs to carry out structured assessments of their long-term mentally ill patients *British Medical Journal* 1995; **311**: 93–98.

12 The Multiaxial Approach to the Primary Care of Schizophrenia

RACHEL JENKINS, Principal Medical Officer, Department of Health, London and MICHAEL SHEPHERD, Emeritus Professor, Institute of Psychiatry, London

SUMMARY

Knowledge of the association between body and mind has existed from early times, and for many centuries, there was no difficulty in conceiving the various ways in which the mind influenced the body in the onset, course and recovery from physical disease. It is really only at the end of the 19th century, when specialisation fragmented medicine into separate and compartmentalised organs and systems, that the mind was effectively separated from the body in medical theory. However, there is a large body of research which emphasises the association between physical and psychological ill health, and between health and social factors, and this paper argues that patients should always be assessed and managed in a multidimensional or multiaxial way instead of addressing only a single physical or psychological axis.

Introduction

This paper describes the advantages of assessing people in a multiaxial way. This is not a new concept—the Church of England's Book of Common Prayer for example takes rather a nice multiaxial approach when it talks of those "in anyways afflicted, or distress in mind, body or estate" in the prayer of *All Conditions of Men*[1]. Earlier philosophers and men of science (see below) also linked body and mind together when assessing physical and emotional wellbeing. Recent medical training however, has tended to promote the `one patient-one diagnosis' model, which cannot do justice to both physical and psychological abnormalities in patients with multiple problems.

Despite this focus, most general practitioners do practice in a very holistic way. This paper brings together some of the history, theory and practice of multiaxial management to put them up for discussion.

Holism and the Multi-axial System of Classification:

Historical background

Knowledge of the association between body and mind has existed from early times: the mind was thought to influence the body via the passions, the imagination and the mental state.

111

(i) Effect of passions

Hippocrates pointed out that fear turns one pale while anger "summons" heat to the head[2]. Galen described how the pulse is generally "altered by quarrels and alarms which suddenly disturb the mind"[3]. Robert Burton, a seventeen th century English physician, observed that "the mind most effectually works upon the body, producing by its passions and perturbations miraculous alterations"[4].

(ii) Effect of imagination

Fienus, a professor of medicine, wrote in 1608 at the University of Louvain (in his De Viribus imaginationis[5]) that through the emotions, the imagination is able to transform the body. "Since the imagination produces change by means of the emotions; and the emotions produce change by means of the natural movement of the heart, and by means of the movement of the humours and the spirits, the imagination does also".

(iii) Effect of mental states

In classical and neoclassical medical theory, mental states were also presumed to cause somatic effects. Hippocrates described how a patient's state of mind influenced his recovery. He wrote "If the soul is burned up... it consumes the body[6]". Robert Burton wrote that the perturbation of the mind could produce "cruel diseases and sometimes death itself"[4].

Early in the history of medicine therefore, there seemed to be no trouble in conceiving the various ways in which the mind influenced the body in the onset, course and recovery from physical disease. Even Descartes, who is often thought to have insisted on the separation of mind and body, joined mind and body together in an intimate interdependency. He argued that the soul is not only "lodged" in the body "as a pilot in a vessel" but is "very closely united to it, and so to speak so intermingled with it that...(soul and body) seem to compose... one whole"[7]. And, in Passions of the Soul[8], he describes a series of states of mind which are the immediate consequences of preceding alterations of the body.

It was only at the end of the 19th century and beginning of the 20th century, when specialisation fragmented medicine into separate and compartmentalised organs and systems, that the mind was firstly effectively separated from the body in most of medical theory. However, a few decades later, psychosomatic medicine arose to reassert these mind-body interactions.

To translate holistic notions into scientifically testable concepts, however, it is necessary to define and examine their components. At the core of this task are the problems associated with classification, a basic issue for both communication and research. In the field of mental disorders the need for an agreed taxonomy has long been recognised and was first tackled systematically by the World Health Organisation in relation to the 9th edition of the International Classification of Disease (ICD). Commenting in the late 1950's on the 'tower of Babel' that characterised the situation world-wide, Stengel entered a plea for the introduction of operational definitions[9]. Shortly afterwards Essen-Möller proposed the adoption of a multi-axial system of diagnosis, advocating one axis for syndromes, sub-divided into symptomatology and 'habitual state', and another for aetiology[10]. Subsequently Zeh urged the addition of an axis for pre-morbid personality[11]. In the early 1960's WHO initiated a series of diagnostic exercises, the first of which was focused on schizophrenia and pointed to the need for a multi-axial approach[12], a conclusion which was endorsed by a later study of childhood disorders[13]. These views were incorporated in the development of the ICD and, later, by the American Psychiatric Association's 3rd edition of the Diagnostic and Statistical Manual[14]. Subsequently, a host of individual workers have explored the application of these ideas to a variety of conditions.

Implications for primary care psychiatry

How do these developments relate to mental illness at the level of primary care? Thirty years ago the survey by Shepherd and his colleagues of 46 general practices demonstrated the very important associations of psychiatric illness and social factors[15]. In the words of the authors, "Emotional disorder in the survey sample was found to be related to a high demand for medical care. Those patients identified as suffering from psychiatric illness attended more frequently and exhibited higher rates of general morbidity and more categories of illness per head than the remainder of the patients consulting their doctors. Furthermore, patients with chronic psychiatric illness were particularly frequent attenders and appeared to constitute a highly vulnerable group from point of view of loss of work and permanent incapacity".

In 1975, a community study by Eastwood[16] found that patients with psychiatric disorders had more physical and psychosomatic conditions than controls. These physical disorders were often multiple, and tended to increase with the severity of the psychiatric disorder. The findings thus confirmed a positive association between physical and psychiatric disorder, with a tendency for clusters of illnesses to occur in some individuals. More recent studies in America[17] and Australia[18], and speakers at the second conference in this series, on the *Prevention of Anxiety and Depression*,[19] have highlighted the close relationship between physical and psychological ill-health[20], and it is clear that people with severe mental illness have a raised mortality, not only from suicide, but also from physical illness[21].

[While the original studies were directed at hospital-based disorders their application to the 'minor' forms of extra-mural morbidity raises several difficulties]. Epidemiological inquiry has demonstrated that the principal ICD rubrics are inadequate for the classification of most psychiatric illnesses including disorders in general practice. As a consequence, in Britain the Research Committee of the Royal College of General Practitioners adapted ICD to construct an International Classification of Health Problems in Primary Care (ICHPPC). To assess the practical value of these schemata Jenkins et al carried out a study exposing a group of senior general practitioners to a set of real-life consultations in the form of videotaped interviews and written case-vignettes covering a range of psychiatric disorders associated with physical, social and personality problems remain[22]. Neither ICD nor ICHPPC enabled the participants to attain a satisfactory level of diagnostic concordance. Their personal formulations were essentially multi-dimensional.

On the basis of the findings derived from this investigation it was possible to construct a classificatory blueprint with 4 axes, namely (i) the psychological phenomena; (2) social problems or supports; (3) personality features comprising illness behaviour and coping abilities; and (4) the physical dimension. This multi-axial schema is summarised in table 12.1:

Table 12.1: *A multiaxial framework of disease*

		Physical	Psychological	Social	Personality	Illness behaviour
I	Antecedent predisposing factors					
II	Direct causes					
III	Pathogenic *~~logical~~ cal* processes caused by the aetiological agent					
IV	Manifestations of the disease					
V	Treatment					
VI	Factors affecting prognosis					

The assessment and management of schizophrenia

How would this multi-axial schema find application to schizophrenia?

(1) *Psychological axis*: Since the diagnosis of schizophrenia is closely linked to psychopathological symptomatology and outcome the clinical presentation of the syndrome calls for separate evaluation.

(2) *Social axis*: In many ways this is the most important axis. It covers several aspects—stresses, personal experiences, and the supports available to help patients cope with their illness and the social disability it incurs. Social support is a major factor in recovery from all illnesses: schizophrenia is no exception. Julian Leff (in chapter one) described how certain social settings (particularly those where 'expressed emotion' is high) can harm people with schizophrenia. Acute life events can also precipitate a relapse unless they are buffered by

appropriate social support. So it is essential to determine whether patients have supportive, reliable friends, colleagues and family, or are socially isolated and lonely. Is it reasonable to presume that social support will be given by their 'nearest and dearest', or should help be arranged via the primary and secondary care teams, social services and the voluntary agencies? If a patient is too ill to personally seek their benefits, they will need an advocate to help them contact and negotiate with the various agencies.

(3) *Personality axis*: The ultimate prognosis in schizophrenia is much better in people whose previous personality was well-integrated or `cyclothymic'. This knowledge may be used to help predict outcome and to develop management programmes for newly-diagnosed patients.

If a patient with schizophrenia becomes ill, either physically or because of psychological deterioration, will he or she consult their GP sooner rather than later, or will they come at all? If the answer is (as often) `no', failsafe mechanisms should be introduced to ensure that such patients receive prompt, appropriate medical care. The capacity of the patient to cope with the demands of daily life also demands careful consideration.

(4) *Physical axis*: The physical correlates of schizophrenia have still to be established. Nonetheless, the patient's physical health should be carefully examined. Is he or she fit and well-nourished, or perhaps vulnerable to infections? Many long-term mentally-ill patients smoke and are at a very high risk of chest diseases. Psychiatric symptomatology can impair their ability to shop, cook and eat a good diet, or take good care of their personal hygiene. For example, a recent newspaper article described a hostel where the occupants were so infected with bed bugs that they all needed blood transfusion. Decisions concerning psychotropic medication also have to be made in relation to the patient's state of mind.

The Care Programme Approach (amended again)

The Care Programme Approach, introduced in England in 1991 embodies these principles of multiaxial assessment, management and review. It arose from major concern that people with severe mental illness were "falling through the safety net of care" into homelessness, prison and even suicide.

The Care Programme Approach involves the assessment of health and social needs, an explicit care plan to meet those needs, allocation of a key worker and a regular review organised by the key worker.

Thus each patient receiving treatment from the mental health service will be allocated a key worker who acts as the focal point of contact for the patient, carer, other community team staff members and the primary health care team. This person is responsible for coordinating the delivery of mental and physical health and social care. He or she will see that regular review and monitoring of the patient's needs and progress occurs.

The community mental health team should invite the primary health care team to participate in the development of the care plan through attendance at care planning and review meetings. If the member of the primary health care team cannot attend, the key worker should seek the views of that team and represent them at the meeting. The key worker should inform the primary health care team of his/her name and telephone number and the care plan which should include arrangements for contacting the community mental health team in an emergency or out of hours.

The Primary Health Care Team should always inform the specialist services of relevant changes in the patient's condition, including frequency and reasons for consultation, expressions of suicidal intent, effects of or changes to medication or other treatment for physical and psychological disorders; should feed in information for care planning purposes and should know how to get hold of the key worker in a crisis.

Conclusion

The evidence briefly presented in this chapter, demonstrates why patients should be assessed and managed in a multidimensional or multiaxial way considering all their needs, instead of addressing only a narrow focus, ie, that he or she has either a physical *or* psychiatric disorder.

Such systems can, par excellence, be applied to schizophrenia, and we have a duty to ensure that medical students are no longer taught the 'one patient—one diagnosis' model.

References

[1] *The Book of Common Prayer* Oxford: OUP

[2] Quoted in Pedro Lain Entralgo *The Therapy of the Word in Classical Antiquity* Ed and trans L J Rather and J M Sharp. New Haven, Connecticut: Yale University Press 1970 pp 162–163.

[3] Quoted in Stanley Jackson Galen—on Mental Disorders. *Journal of the History of Behavioural Sciences* 1969 **5**, 366.

[4] Robert Burton 1621. *The Anatomy of Melancholy* ed A R Shillets, London, George Bell and Sons 1893, Vol 1 p 288.

[5] Quoted in L J Rather. Thomas Fierus (1567–1631) Dialectical Investigation of the Imagination as Cause and Cure of Bodily Disease *Bulletin of the History of Medicine* 1967 **41**, 349–67.

[6] Quoted in P L Entralgo. *The Therapy of the Word in Classical Antiquity*. Ed and Trans L J Rather and J M Sharp. New Haven, Connecticut: Yale University Press 1970 p 161.

[7] E S Haldane and G R T Ross (Translators). *Descartes, The Philosophical Works* New York: Dover, 1955 Vol 1, p 120.

[8] E S Haldane and G R T Ross (Translators). *Descartes, The Philosophical Works*. New York, Dover, 1955 Vol 1, p 344–375.

[9] Stengel E 1959 Classification of mental disorders Bulletin or World Health Organisation 21, 601–663.

[10] Essen-Möller E 1961 On classification of mental disorders Acta Psychiatrica Scandinavica 37, 199–126.

[11] Zeh W 1962 Bemerkungen zu einem Klassifikationsverschlag der psychischem Storungen von Erik Essen-Möller, Lund.

[12] Shepherd M, Brooke E M, Cooper S E and LinT 1968 An experiment approach to psychiatric diagnosis: an informational study Acta psychiatrica Scandvianica Supplementum 201 Munksgaard, Copenhagen.

[13] Rutter M, Shalfer D, Shepherd M 1973. An evaluation of the proposal for a multiaxial classification of child psychiatric disorders Psychological Medicine 3, 244–250.

[14] Regier D A, Booke J P, Burns B J, Clare A W, Gulbiat W, Luplain M, Siter R L, Williams S B W, and Woud M 1982. A proposed classification of social problems and psycholigcal symptoms for inclusion in a classification of healtg problems Ch 11 In Psychosocial Factors affecting Health (ed Macklipkin and Karel Kupka) pp 153–184 Praeger, New York.

[15] Shepherd M, Cooper B, Brown A C, Kactan G W. *Psychiatric illness in general practice.* Oxford University Press, London 1966.

[16] Eastwood M R. *The relation between physical and mental illness.* Toronto: University of Toronto Press 1975.

[17] Kessler L G, Burns B J, Sharpio S, Tischler G L, George L K, Hough R L, Bodison D and Miller R H. Psychiatric diagnosis of medical service users: Evidence from the Epidemiologic Catchment Area Program. *American Journal of Public Health* 1987 **77**, 18–24.

[18] Andrews A, Schonell M and Tennant C. The Relationship between physical, psychological and social morbidity in a suburban community. *American Journal of Epidemiology* 1977 **106**, 324–9.

[19] *Prevention of Depression and Anxiety—the role of the practice team.* Edited by Jenkins R, Newton J and Young R. London, HMSO 1991.

[20] Maguire G P and Granville-Grossman K L. Physical illness in psychiatric patients. *British Journal of Psychiatry* 1968 **114**, 1365–9.

[21] Fox A J Goldblatt P O. *Longitudinal Study—Sociodemographic Mortality Differential.* L S No 1, 1971–1975. London: HMSO 1982.

[22] Jenkins R, Smeeton N and Shepherd M. 1988. Classification of mental disorder in primary care. *Psychological Medicine, Monograph Supplement* 12. Cambridge University Press 1988.